Eating on the Run

Third Edition

Evelyn Tribole, MS, RD

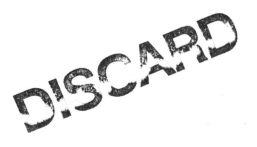

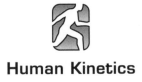

Human Kinetics

Library of Congress Cataloging-in-Publication Data

Tribole, Evelyn, 1959-
  Eating on the run / by Evelyn Tribole.--3rd ed.
    p. cm.
Includes bibliographical references and index.
  ISBN 0-7360-4608-9 (softcover)
1. Nutrition. 2. Quick and easy cookery. 3. Convenience foods.
4. Time management. I. Title.
RA784.T75 2004
  613.2--dc22

                                                                  2003016272

ISBN: 0-7360-4608-9

The Web addresses cited in this text were current as of August 26, 2003, unless otherwise noted.

Acquisitions Editor: Martin Barnard; **Managing Editor:** Wendy McLaughlin; **Assistant Editor:** Kim Thoren; **Copyeditor:** Karen Bojda; **Proofreader:** Sue Fetters; **Indexer:** Betty Frizzéll; **Permission Manager:** Toni Harte; **Graphic Designer:** Andrew Tietz; **Graphic Artist:** Tara Welsch; **Photo Manager:** Dan Wendt; **Cover Designer:** Keith Blomberg; **Photographer (cover):** Dan Wendt; **Art Manager:** Kareema McLendon; **Illustrator:** Brian McElwain; **Printer:** United Graphics

Human Kinetics books are available at special discounts for bulk purchase. Special editions or book excerpts can also be created to specification. For details, contact the Special Sales Manager at Human Kinetics.

Printed in the United States of America   10 9 8 7 6 5 4 3 2 1

Human Kinetics
Web site: www.HumanKinetics.com

United States: Human Kinetics
P.O. Box 5076
Champaign, IL 61825-5076
800-747-4457
e-mail: humank@hkusa.com

Canada: Human Kinetics
475 Devonshire Road Unit 100
Windsor, ON N8Y 2L5
800-465-7301 (in Canada only)
e-mail: orders@hkcanada.com

Europe: Human Kinetics
107 Bradford Road
Stanningley
Leeds LS28 6AT, United Kingdom
+44 (0) 113 255 5665
e-mail: hk@hkeurope.com

Australia: Human Kinetics
57A Price Avenue
Lower Mitcham, South Australia 5062
08 8277 1555
e-mail: liaw@hkaustralia.com

New Zealand: Human Kinetics
Division of Sports Distributors NZ Ltd.
P.O. Box 300 226 Albany
North Shore City
Auckland
0064 9 448 1207
e-mail: blairc@hknewz.com

To Krystin and Connor

CONTENTS

ACKNOWLEDGMENTS

No book is truly written alone and therefore I am grateful for the support and help from all of my clients and patients, who have taught me the realistic side of nutrition—the art of eating with pleasure while honoring health and time constraints: Elyse Resch, MS, RD, FADA, and Nancy Clark, MS, RD, for technical review and comments; Jenn Hanlin, a terrific research assistant in a pinch; to all my book publicists past and future, as they are the unsung heroes of book promotion; David Hale Smith, literary agent extraordinaire and a great sounding board; Krystin Tribole, a meticulous data entry assistant and practical proofreader; Human Kinetics Publishing staff—Martin Barnard, acquisitions editor, for his patience and gentle persistence, and Wendy McLaughlin, my editor for her cheerful attitude, which was truly appreciated during the editing process. Most of all I would like to thank my family who gave me the space and time to update this book.

INTRODUCTION

When I wrote the second edition of *Eating on the Run*, almost 10 years ago, e-mail and the Internet as we know them were in a fledgling stage, not easily accessed by regular folks. In 2001, an estimated 1.4 trillion (yes, trillion) messages originated from businesses alone, according to the *Wall Street Journal*. Employees spend an average of 49 minutes a day clearing out e-mail, and for top management it's nearly four hours a day. Today, even e-mail is too slow for some; now we have "instant messaging." Cell phones were once a rarity. Now it's rare if a person doesn't have a cell phone, and they are so pervasive that new laws outlaw their use while driving. Yet in spite of these advances in technology, we are busier than ever and more vulnerable to unhealthy eating.

There are now many opportunities to eat 24 hours a day, seven days a week—from gas stations to bookstores. While this appears to be a helpful trend, it may be just the opposite. We are now living in what some researchers call a toxic food environment. This concept explains the unprecedented way food has come to be sold, advertised, and prepared in the last decade and the way the food industry competes for market share (also known as "share of stomach"). All this marketing clamor is not for selling broccoli on every corner.

According to the U.S. Department of Agriculture (USDA) Economic Research Service (ERS), food manufacturers spend $7 billion in advertising, but only 2 percent of this advertising money was spent on fruits, vegetables, grains, and beans combined. The ERS also found that the foods with the highest advertising intensity are the ones we overeat as judged by national nutritional recommendations. One of the most notable food marketing trends is supersizing: extra large drinks, meal portions, you name it.

Paradoxically, as a nation we have more nutritional information now than ever before, but we are stumbling nutritionally. New food labeling laws enacted in the last decade require calories and key nutrient information to be provided on nearly every packaged food. Many food companies have additional nutritional information on their Web sites. So why are we having such a tough time in this age of technology and instant access to information? Clearly, it's not that we lack nutritional knowledge; rather, it's often what we do at critical moments. We seem to be juggling more items on our life agendas. When forced to choose between meeting a deadline or eating, sometimes the deadline wins. For example, in a time crunch at lunch, do you choose to eat or run errands, only to suffer ravenous hunger and succumb to a super combo meal with big, big fries on the way back to the office? Or perhaps you grab lunch and eat mindlessly at your desk while finishing a project, only to realize too late that you overate.

In my nutrition counseling practice I see clients for a variety of reasons; many have eating disorders, and others want to eat more healthfully, lower their cholesterol, or improve their sport performance. Although my patients are diverse, one striking commonality is the challenge of how and what they eat when pressed for time. Patients have sat in my office with audibly growling stomachs because they did not have time to eat a meal or snack! Nourishing your body needs to become a nonnegotiable priority, regardless of how hectic your life is or how much multitasking you must do. My clients are my best teachers when it comes to practical, real-world nutrition advice. In this third edition of *Eating on the Run,* I share with you the tried and true strategies that I recommend to my clients and use myself, as I have become busier too, juggling a nutrition counseling practice, family, and travel for speaking engagements and media appearances.

This edition includes many changes and updates to help you navigate the world of around-the-clock access to food in your busy life. The good news is that there are more possibilities for getting a healthier bite or meal—if you know where and what to get. For example, a quick latte at the ubiquitous Starbucks at an airport or bookstore provides one third or more of your calcium requirements, depending on the size of your drink.

Part I discusses basic nutrition facts everyone needs to know, plus tips for fitting your meals into a jam-packed schedule and for healthy, speedy grocery shopping. Part II deals with how to eat right on the go—at work, in your car, at the airport. Part III guides you through the mountains of information regarding diets, supplements, and making quick and nutritious meals for your busy family. In Part IV you'll find fantastic, tasty, quick and even one-minute meals and advice on surviving the holidays. I've also included updated nutrition information for common fast foods, additional resources, tips for vegans, and eating and ordering ethnic cuisine. You can read *Eating on the Run* cover to cover, or you can just zoom in on the chapters that are most relevant to you. We're all busy, but we all have to eat. The trick is knowing how to do it right for your life.

PART I

Nutrition in a Nutshell

CHAPTER 1

Food Facts for Busy People

What do you do about eating during a critical time crunch? Most of the busy clients that I work with have a lot of nutritional knowledge and value their health. But the main challenge, over and over again, is how they act on that knowledge at critical moments. Here's an illustrative example.

A physician decided at 11:00 P.M. that surgery was needed for a patient who was admitted to the emergency room. When the surgeon notified the spouse that he was operating in an hour (it would take that long to prep the patient and the room), the spouse asked, "Have you had dinner?" He replied, " No." To his surprise, the spouse insisted that the surgeon have something to eat for the midnight surgery, as he had not eaten *since* lunch. Clearly, nutrition knowledge did not keep this doctor from his meal; it was his very long, hectic day. But he neglected to make time to eat even a snack.

It is a challenge to make feeding your body a nonnegotiable priority. But consider it a vaccine against overeating and brain drain. Do not underestimate the power of primal hunger, especially when combined with fatigue and stress. Here are some common scenarios I see play out time after time:

- A business executive polishes off three doughnuts at a morning meeting. It isn't lack of nutrition knowledge that does him in. Skipping breakfast makes him vulnerable.

- A sales rep skips lunch to squeeze in one more client appointment, only to succumb to ravenous hunger at dinner at a Mexican restaurant by eating an entire basket of tortilla chips.

- In a frenzied family, two kids have dueling soccer practices until early evening. Mom or dad drives through a local fast-food window and orders a round of combo meals for the family.

- A college student whose evening class goes from 6 to 9 P.M. postpones dinner until he gets back home. You can probably guess what happens: pizza.

- An attorney eats only one meal, dinner, to save time (and calories, so she thinks) yet cannot understand why she is often fatigued and experiences brain drain in the afternoon.

Do any of these examples sound familiar to you? What do your own experiences with missing meals or going too long without eating demonstrate to you? Your own experiences can be powerful learning tools if you take the time to examine them. Keep in mind that one missed meal is not going to make or break your health, but a recurring pattern of chaotic eating can certainly have an impact.

In my counseling practice, I've noticed that fewer and fewer people actually cook. My clients are often embarrassed to admit that they seldom cook or that they don't like cooking. After a long, hectic day, the last thing you may want to do is cook a meal. Fine! Don't apologize. You are busy—end of story. The problem is that many people fall into the trap of all or none: "If I can't eat perfectly healthfully, I'll just get a combo meal at the drive-through." "I'll have a pizza delivered." "I'll just microwave a bag of popcorn and call it dinner." Nutrition myths also can keep people stuck in bad eating habits. Let's look at a few common myths.

NUTRITION MYTHS

There are several common myths about eating fast food, eating at restaurants, late-night meals, and so on. Let's clear up some of this misinformation.

If you eat fast food, you are doomed to poor health.

While a classic fast-food meal can easily be loaded with too many fat calories and too much sodium, fast food can be a good option. Yes, you read that correctly! For example, if you are squeezed for time and need to choose between skipping lunch or drive-through fast food, choosing a healthy fast-food option can be beneficial. All too often people eschew fast food because they think it's too unhealthy but then end up attacking the vending machine because they get too hungry. It is important to figure out the choices that are healthiest.

Eating out at restaurants too often is unhealthy.

While it's true that the typical restaurant meal has 1,000 to 2,000 calories, even without the bread basket, beverage, or dessert, there are nevertheless some much better options that taste fabulous. In fact, some of my healthiest meals come from restaurants! Of course, it helps to know how to navigate the menu and break free from the clean-plate club (of which many of my clients are ardent members). Chapter 4 is devoted to restaurant eating.

You have to cook or eat home-cooked meals to be healthy.

There are more healthy "no-cook" options than ever before. One of my favorite confessions is that I don't like to cook during weekdays. This revelation often shocks my clients because I've written three cookbooks. And I absolutely dislike cleaning up the dishes. The truth of the matter is that during the week—between my work schedule, my kids' activities, and so forth—cooking can be a real chore. I felt validated by Frances Mayes' memoir *Under the Tuscan Sun,* in which Mayes, a college professor from San Francisco, describes renovating a farmhouse in Italy. The author describes with great flair the joy of food preparation while in Italy (usually during summer breaks), from growing and harvesting olives to making olive oil to creating leisurely Italian feasts from the local homegrown bounty. But when she enters into the chaos of her work schedule in California, cooking reverts to a survival chore rather than a pleasurable pursuit.

Snacking is unhealthy and leads to weight gain.

Snacking can be quite healthy and can actually prevent overeating. Snacking is so important that I devote the next chapter to its benefits and pitfalls. One major pitfall can be mindless nibbling, which is not based on hunger.

If you eat late, after 8:00 P.M., you will gain weight.

Your body does not punch a time clock: "It's 8:00 P.M., time to start making fat!" This is one of the biggest food myths I encounter. Your body orchestrates fulfilling its needs like a great symphony, based on its current biological state. If you finish work at 6:30 P.M. and head to the gym for a workout, you could easily arrive home at 8:00 quite hungry for dinner. In this situation, your body biologically needs to eat, and it's quite reasonable to eat dinner!

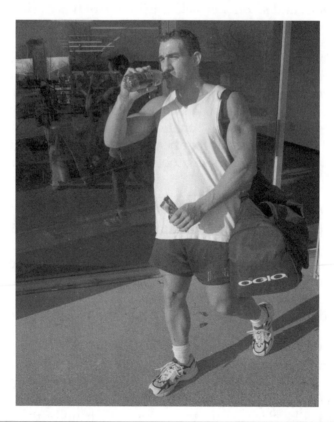

Snacking is a great way to get the nutrition you need while enjoying a multitude of activities.

Being busy leads to poor nutrition and bad eating habits.

Not at all. But when you are wiped out and hungry, it's all too easy to give in to any food resembling a meal, such as a double cheeseburger or a sausage pizza.

It takes a lot of time to eat healthfully.

This is the perception of many Americans. The truth is that it doesn't take much time at all to eat healthfully. You need to be prepared, however, or it's all too easy to succumb to your eating environment. It doesn't take any longer to grill fish than to grill a steak. In fact, fish is faster. It doesn't take any longer to heat a healthy frozen meal than an unhealthy one. It doesn't take any longer to order a vegetable-topped pizza than a pepperoni-topped one. You get the idea.

You have to be a nutrition whiz or dietitian to know how to eat healthfully.

The basic tenets of healthy eating have not changed. Reams of research show how and why specific foods confer health benefits, but the basic principles that you need to eat your vegetables and so forth haven't changed. Let's look at these basic nutritional principles.

NUTRITION BOOT CAMP

Nutritional knowledge is very helpful as long you don't beat yourself up with it. I've worked with too many brilliant people who feel incredible guilt about their food choices. The truth is that food guilt is never helpful! It's okay to regret a food choice. Learn from the event that triggered the eating experience. Then let it go and move on. While nutritional *knowledge* is not the critical, factor when in a time crunch, it can be very helpful when making food choices in a hurry. Enter nutrition boot camp. I'll keep this short and sweet, just the basics for now.

Hitting the Nutrition Target

A client of mine who was a financial planner strongly believed in having a target when establishing financial goals: "You've got to have a target, or how will you know if you've arrived?" This principle can be used with nutrition as well. One of the easiest targets to use is the Food Guide Pyramid. This might seem very basic, but most Americans miss the target in every food group! A recent USDA report showed that, in a nutshell, we're eating too many of the things that contribute to poor health (fat, cholesterol, and calories) but falling short of critical nutrients (folic acid and calcium). Americans are not meeting even the minimum recommendations for the Pyramid's five major food groups. Are you getting at least the minimum?

- **Grains** (preferably whole grains)—Six servings each day. One serving is generally one-half cup of rice, cereal, or pasta, or one slice of bread or one tortilla.

- **Vegetables**—Three servings each day. This is the equivalent of eating one and one-half cups of cooked vegetables a day. They don't have to be three different vegetables, just three servings' worth, although variety is certainly helpful.
- **Fruits**—Two servings a day, which is one piece of medium fruit, one-half cup of cut-up or canned fruit, or six ounces of fruit juice.
- **Protein**—Four to nine ounces a day of high-protein foods such as fish, meat, or chicken. These count as one ounce of protein: one egg, one-half cup of cooked beans, two tablespoons of peanut butter.
- **Calcium-rich foods**—Three servings daily. One serving is one cup of milk, yogurt, calcium-fortified orange juice, or one and one-half ounces of natural cheese.

The Nutrition 6-5-4-3-2 Countdown

The nutrition countdown is a simple way to remember the minimum servings needed from each food group. The numbers are easy to remember and give you a target for each day. For my financially minded friends, this is the equivalent of the allocation method of investing. You just need to make sure that you make your distributions in the right amounts and you will have a balanced portfolio, that is, a balanced diet.

6 servings of whole grains

5 servings of fruits and vegetables, combined; more is even better

4 to 9 ounces of lean protein; remember that this includes beans and nuts, too

3 servings of calcium-rich foods

2 servings of fish each week

I went beyond the Food Guide Pyramid and added fish twice a week because the health benefits are so profound. I talk more about that in chapter 8, "Eating for Health and Longevity."

"Making Peace" With Food

I like to simplify the Food Pyramid by aiming for the minimum goals and giving you an idea of what these look like on your plate. I use this model of healthful eating to help my clients plan on a meal-by-meal basis. Optimally there is a grain source, some type of plant food (fruit or vegetables), and some protein. This model helps to promote balanced eating and satiety. I also like that the plate resembles a peace sign: Food should be our ally, not the enemy!

HEALTHY EATING TENETS

When it comes to tenets of healthful eating, moderation and variety certainly make sense, but they're not very tangible. I find the best way to give these noble concepts meaning is to examine your eating over a week to see how you truly are doing. In fact, most nutrition guidelines are intended as an average over a week's time. One snack, one meal, one day does not make or break your health. Remember that progress, not perfection, is what counts.

Quality and Diversity

Quality food choices mean that you get the most bang for the nutritional buck. Quality choices include higher-fiber foods; healthy fats such as nuts, seeds, avocados, olive oil, and canola oil; whole grains; low-fat dairy products; and lean protein sources.

Diversity is a key concept for investing; the same principle holds true for eating. Yet how often do you get stuck eating the same old thing for breakfast or lunch? Certainly this is an easy way to eat; it requires no thinking. But the down side is that not only can this be boring, but you might be placing yourself in a nutritional rut. Variety ensures you get the 50-odd nutrients and phytochemicals (natural health-promoting compounds found in plant foods, many of which are still being discovered) that you need.

Try simple changes to diversify your eating. For example, vary the cereals you eat, mix them, or rotate brands. This helps you get different types of fiber that have different benefits. For example, oats and oat bran are rich in soluble fiber, which promotes heart health by lowering cholesterol. Whole wheat and wheat bran are high in insoluble fiber, which promotes intestinal health. Change the type of juice you drink. With so many different real fruit juices and 100 percent juice blends to choose from, there's no reason to settle on just one.

Creating Time to Eat

If you have just 60 seconds, you have time to eat nutritiously. Remember, there is no nutritional law that requires you to sit down to a hot meal. Tight schedules call for nutritional survival, which means having a "nutritional 911" plan ready to go. It doesn't have to be a rigid plan; it can be as simple as throwing a couple of energy bars in your briefcase. Most people meticulously plan what they will do in a day, from business meetings to car tune-ups to golf games to manicures. Many people have planning down to an art using computers and PDAs—except when it comes to feeding their bodies.

For some reason, when I mention the "p" word—planning—to clients, they grimace. The barriers come up and the excuses fly for why they don't plan their eating the same way they plan their daily schedule, even though they pride themselves on their organized appointment books. Some typical excuses may sound familiar to you:

"I have to wait until I'm hungry."

"I don't know where I'll be."

"I don't have time to plan."

"I don't know how long my meetings will last."
"I'm in my car all day."

Don't worry. Your plan for feeding your body does not have to be rigid. Actually, it should be quite the opposite: It must have flexibility built in. But you do need a foundation from which to build.

Identifying Eating Opportunities   It's important to find time to eat, be it a snack, a mini-meal, or a full meal. Even when they're chasing deadlines or catching planes, most people have an idea of what the upcoming day will be like. Even if chaos seems to be your norm or you feel like a slave to your appointment book, here's how you can make sure you have an opportunity to eat.

Ask yourself how you can best fit eating into your schedule. Some days it may seem impossible. If so, could you combine eating with another activity? For instance, you could eat while

- walking to your car, train, plane, or classroom;
- getting ready for work, school, or a meeting;
- driving or riding;
- working at your desk; or
- killing time between appointments.

It is ideal to sit down for 20 minutes and do nothing but eat and savor the food (mindful eating). But when you are in a time crunch, eating is a matter of survival. *It is better to fuel your body in a less-than-ideal setting than to go without eating.*

Timing is another factor when planning opportunities to eat. Be sure that you go no longer than five hours without eating. Why five hours? Your body's primary energy source is glucose (as in blood sugar). Glucose is stored in your liver as glycogen and normally runs out in two to six hours (depending on what and how much you last ate). If you do not replenish liver glycogen with food (carbohydrates), your body is running on empty and will to resort to creative fueling by breaking down muscle tissue to convert to glucose or using protein *from* your diet for energy rather than for its prime use in rebuilding muscle, enzymes, and hormones.

Planning Meal by Meal   The most difficult eating times seem to be breakfast and lunch, yet dinner is the most challenging to plan because it seems too time-consuming to many people.

- **Breakfast.** Don't leave home without it. Numerous studies show the benefits of eating breakfast. If you are not used to eating early, you may just need a little time to get adjusted. A general rule of thumb is to eat within two hours of waking or rising. The best approach is to start simple. There's nothing wrong with leftovers, or good old cereal and milk is easy and quick.

If for some reason even this seems too overwhelming, make sure you graze on a morning snack, such as a piece of whole-grain toast with peanut butter. (For more speedy meal ideas, see chapter 13, which gives 40 mini-meals that take 60 seconds or less to make.)

↗ **Lunch.** Lunch hour? What's that? Many of my industrious clients work straight through lunch. "Looks good on the corporate resume," they say. If they do decide to use their "lunch hour," it is not usually for eating but for running errands. In fact, a survey by Datamonitor, an independent market analysis firm, reported on the demise of the traditional lunch hour throughout Europe and the United States. The average lunchtime has shrunk to 36 minutes. If finding time for lunch is a problem, try packing a lunch or throwing some wholesome snacks into your briefcase. Keep healthy grazing foods stocked in the office kitchen, your car, or your backpack or briefcase. (Grazing and fast food are addressed in upcoming chapters.)

According to a consumer survey conducted by Tupperware, two out of three workers (66 percent) in the United States take their lunch to work. A brown-bag lunch has the advantage of being there, readily available for you to graze on all day long if you don't have time for a real lunch break. When possible, I highly recommend eating away from your desk or workplace for the following reasons:

- It helps clear the mind.
- It gives you a rest that enhances your productivity.
- It's a good stress breaker.
- It's more enjoyable and satisfying.
- It makes you a more conscious eater.

On days when you are rushed, you may try eating alone rather than with coworkers. Take a book with you; that's usually a polite cue that you want to be alone, and generally you will not be disturbed.

↗ **Dinner.** This is the most troublesome meal for many people to plan. After a long day, just thinking about dinner can seem exhausting. You come home and gaze into the refrigerator or cupboards, as if waiting for something to magically appear. You finally decide (a feat in itself) that spaghetti sounds good, but you find your cupboards are bare—and your stomach is rumbling. By this time, you settle for anything. Tonight it's popcorn for dinner. Does this scenario sound familiar?

Day after day, waiting for inspiration (which is not likely to come when you are fatigued)—not only is this routine tiresome, but it wastes your precious time. One solution is what I call the five-in-five approach. This technique is the most effective and easiest to use. Since planning dinner was always such an obstacle, I routinely began to have my clients plan five dinners (only the main entree, which is usually the major stumbling block) in my office. Meanwhile, I was secretly timing them. When they finished planning, I would announce how long it took. On the average, it took five minutes or less to plan five meals. Easy! And to think that they would often waste 10 minutes or more daily trying to come up with something to eat for dinner. Why plan five meals rather than a whole week (seven meals)? It has been my experience that, between leftovers and eating out, five meals easily stretch into a week's worth of eating.

By the way, please do *not* feel obligated to always having chicken on Monday, chili on Tuesday, and so on; that would be too rigid. On a given day, just select any meal from your plan. Of course, you must make sure that you have all the ingredients on hand. Optimally, you shop for groceries based on the list of meals you have planned.

One benefit from the five-in-five technique is how much better you feel when you arrive home and have an idea of what is for dinner. You will feel calmer and less stressed, and you won't have to make any more last minute dashes to the store.

It's easy to grab five minutes to plan meals. Do it while waiting

- for a meeting to start,
- in line at the bank,
- for an appointment, or
- anywhere!

Once you have created your meal list, post it somewhere convenient. To save more time, try making a master list of all meals you are willing to prepare (and eat). Use the master list to plan the five meals. It doesn't require any thinking, just choosing!

CHAPTER 2

Grazing on the Go

"I have no time to eat, so I just drink coffee all day long until I get home."—Television news reporter

Time, or rather the lack of it, is the most common obstacle to eating that my clients disclose to me. My usual response is, "Do you have 60 seconds?" I have not yet met a person who says they can't spare one minute, yet that's all it really takes. In this chapter, you'll learn about grazing, a simple way to bring nutrition into your life on the run.

SKIPPING MEALS

Let's look at the problems of skipping meals or going so long without eating that it's like a mini-fast. One of the biggest consequences is what I call primal hunger. That's when your body gets so hungry that anything goes: all honorable intentions about health fly out the window. Your body is hardwired for survival, and if you go too long without eating, it goes into survival mode by sending you on a food quest. Although no true famine threatens your survival, your cells do not know that there are 24-hour grocery stores and fast-food restaurants on every corner! The bottom line is that if you go too long without eating, you are likely to eat too much at the next opportunity. Therefore, skipping breakfast, or any meal for that matter, will catch up with you. In fact, adding a timely snack or grazing is like a vaccine to prevent overeating.

Consider these other consequences of meal skipping:

▰ **Poor performance.** Meal skippers don't perform as well. They accomplish less work, are physically less steady, and are slower at making decisions.

▰ **Brain drain.** The brain's exclusive fuel, glucose, is compromised within four to six hours if you have not eaten. That's because the glucose stored in the liver as glycogen, runs out during this time period. The liver is like a traffic cop for blood sugar. When blood glucose dips too low, the liver converts glycogen into glucose and releases it into the blood. But if its glycogen has been depleted, the body has to turn to less efficient fueling methods.

11

◢ **Calorie loading.** Calorie loading easily occurs if you eat just one meal a day (typically dinner). Eating just one large meal tends to overwhelm your body with calories that it does not need at that moment. It's like plugging all the appliances in your house into one socket. Even though the entire electrical system can handle all the appliances, if they are concentrated on just one circuit, you'll blow a fuse. It is better to spread the nutrient load.

Despite the known side effects of skipping meals, it's easy to get caught in the trap of doing without. Here are some common reasons that people skip meals:

Breakfast: Getting up too late, not feeling hungry, nothing to eat

Lunch: Tied up in meetings, running errands, forgetting to bring lunch, forgetting to bring cash, behind on project deadlines

Dinner: Meeting after work, evening aerobics class, arriving home late

Another common problem is stress. People often become so focused on a project or so stressed and overwhelmed that they truly don't experience hunger. There is a reason for this. Stress hormones can blunt hunger. And since time is precious, it's easy to postpone eating. The next thing you know, it's dinner time, and you haven't even had lunch.

The breakfast skippers that I work with often say, "I'm not hungry in the morning." If you're the same way, it is likely that you have conditioned your body over a number of years not to be hungry. When hunger is ignored often enough, you don't feel it! Nonetheless, your body still needs to be fed.

Weight Loss and Breakfast

What's the relationship between weight loss and breakfast? That's what researchers from the National Weight Control Registry (NWCR) wanted to know. The NWCR was created in 1994 to research the characteristics and behaviors of people who have been successful at losing weight and keeping it off in the long term. To qualify, individuals must have maintained a weight loss of at least 30 pounds for over a year. In this particular breakfast study, the nearly 3,000 people surveyed had lost 70 pounds and kept it off for six years on average. The researchers found a compelling trend: a very high proportion (78 percent) of these weight-loss maintainers ate breakfast every day of the week. The researchers concluded that eating breakfast is a characteristic of successful weight-loss maintainers and may be a key factor in their success.

A lack of time is a popular excuse to skip meals. Who has time to eat, really? Remember that you don't need to sit down to three big meals. Instead, you can eat fast, nutritious mini-meals, especially when time is fleeting. For example, breakfast is just a matter of having something to eat in the morning, even if you have to wait until you get to the office. A quick mini-breakfast could be as easy a glass of orange juice and a cup of milk—it takes all of 19 seconds to prepare. (Yes, I timed it!) In fact, when I encourage clients to eat *something* in the morning, I give this simple 19-second example. They often respond with a look of relief. This is how I introduce them to grazing.

GRAZING

Grazing is simply eating small mini-meals or snacks throughout the day. You can eat whenever and wherever you want—at home or on the job, at any time of the day. This flexibility can fit into anyone's schedule. When grazing, you are only one bite away from your next meal. Although the "graze craze" may sound trendy, it actually resembles the original eating patterns of our gatherer ancestors over two million years ago.

Benefits of Grazing

Besides the timesaving benefit of grazing, many studies have demonstrated amazing nutritional merits of grazing. Grazing is also known as nibbling or spreading the nutrient load. Here are some of the payoffs that grazing has to offer:

1. **Lower cholesterol and healthier arteries.** A classic study reported in the *New England Journal of Medicine* in 1989 demonstrated that a grazing pattern of eating resulted in lower blood cholesterol. The subjects were divided into two different groups and given *identical* diets. The only difference was *how* they ate. The "nibbling" group ate their food divided into 17 snacks a day. The "meal" group ate their food in three meals. The researchers concluded that a nibbling diet, or increased meal frequency, could play a role in the prevention of heart disease. But eating 17 times a day is too extreme for most people!

Fortunately, several newer studies have shown that grazing as few as four small meals a day can lower cholesterol. In a particularly promising study from London, researchers demonstrated for the first time that the arteries of smokers experience an actual protective affect from grazing. Those who ate more frequently had significantly less risk of symptomatic atherosclerosis.

2. **Brainpower.** The results of a 1990 study by Kanarek and Swinney illustrate the brainpower of timely snacking or grazing. Students given fruited yogurt for an afternoon snack had a significant increase in mental performance compared with those who had only a diet soda. (The researchers measured mental performance by giving a battery of tests that included memory tests, math reasoning, reading, and attention span.)

Similar results were shown in another recent study in which a midmorning snack was added. Those who ate a midmorning snack had improved mood and memory compared with those who ate no morning snack. Think about how often you try to tide yourself over with a diet beverage or a cup of coffee. You may be temporarily fooling your stomach, but it catches up with you. Coffee drinkers, could I interest you in a latte instead?

3. **Weight control.** Ironically, despite the metabolic benefits of grazing, many people thinking of snacking as no-no. They fear that it may lead to gaining weight, when it can do just the opposite. A recent review of 12 studies on the impact of snacking on weight showed that snacking does not adversely affect weight control and can actually be helpful.

More often than not, when I ask clients when they experience hunger or feel most vulnerable to eating, they reply, "In the afternoon." When I ask what they do about this urge, the typical reply is "nothing": they play "meal martyr" by waiting long hours until their next meal. For example, if you have lunch at noon but you work late and don't get home until 8 P.M., your body is running on empty. As a consequence, by the time you have an opportunity to eat, you are more likely to gorge.

In fact one study showed that dividing food intake into five eating occasions resulted in a flatter profile of hunger throughout the day compared to those spreading their calories into three meals. (Both groups had the same amount of daily calories) The researchers concluded that less built-up hunger at mealtimes helps to prevent gorging at meals.

How can simply changing the frequency of eating confer all these benefits? The prevailing theory is that by eating smaller amounts of food more often, less insulin is released. Insulin is a powerful hormone that turns on the enzyme that makes cholesterol. When less insulin is released, the body makes less cholesterol. Similarly, spreading the nutrient load results in a more sustained release of carbohydrate, which helps keep the blood sugar level steady. A steady blood sugar level improves memory, increases energy, and prevents ravenous hunger, which can lead to overeating.

Pitfalls of Grazing

With all the compelling benefits of grazing, how could there be a down side? The biggest grazing downfall is the trap of mindless eating, or what I refer to as "eating amnesia." We've become a multitasking generation. Why get only one thing accomplished when you can do at least two tasks at a time? When it comes to eating, this can be a problem, whether you are eating and reading, eating and watching TV, or eating and checking e-mail. This paired eating is not a problem once in a while, especially if it's the only time you can squeeze in eating, which is better than skipping a meal. But chronically eating while doing another activity can lead to eating amnesia: you forget what or, more likely, how much you have eaten. Most people have trouble remembering what they ate for their last full meal, let alone their last bite of this or spoonful of that.

Two Days of Grazing at a Glance

Day 1: Fast and Furious   Here's how you could graze on a fly-by-the-seat-of-your-pants day, when you hit the local eateries, vending machines, and coffee shops. As you rush through your day, try these choices instead of the Extra Value Meals at McDonald's.

Morning	16-oz. latte (with fat-free milk)
	Whole wheat bagel with light cream cheese
	Fruit cup
Midmorning	McDonald's Fruit 'n Yogurt Parfait with granola
Lunch	Subway Honey Mustard Ham (6-inch)
	Veggie Delite salad with fat-free dressing
	Iced tea
Afternoon	Small bag of pretzels from vending machine
Dinner	Meal at Koo Koo Roo:
	Fruit salad
	Steamed vegetables
	Baked beans
	Chicken (without skin)

Day 2: 9 to 5   Here's what a typical day of grazing could look like on a calmer day. These five eating occasions require no cooking, except for heating up a frozen pizza.

Morning	1 cup raisin bran cereal, topped with banana slices
	1 cup milk
Midmorning	Apple and peanut butter
Lunch	Turkey sandwich on whole wheat bread with lettuce, tomato, low-fat cheese, and mustard
	1 small bag baby carrots
	1 pear
Afternoon	Instant cup of bean soup and whole wheat crackers
Dinner	1/2 frozen Wolfgang Puck vegetable pizza
	Bag of prepared salad with Italian dressing, Parmesan cheese, and walnuts

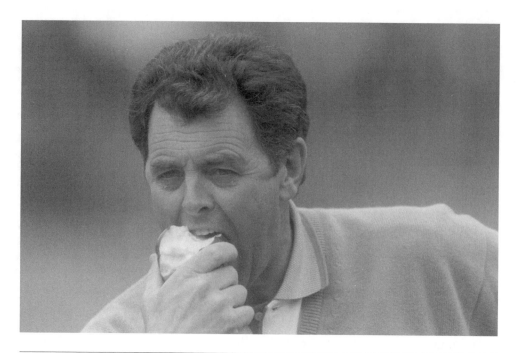

Apples are great grazing foods.

Mindless nibblers start out innocently with little tastes here and there, but the next thing they know, a whole box of crackers or cookies is gone. Perhaps only when they feel their fingertips scrape against the bottom of the package do they realize the quantity consumed while their minds were somewhere else.

To avoid going down the mindless eating path, try these approaches to become a more conscious eater:

1. When possible, sit and savor. Remember that when you are grazing, the smaller amounts of food that you are eating won't take as long to eat as a traditional meal.

2. Divvy out your snacks. For example, instead of eating from an endless box of crackers, allocate a reasonable amount, say five crackers. Put them in a baggie or on a plate. You can nibble on them throughout the day, and when the package is empty, you will know what and how much you ate.

3. Keep a mental record of what you are eating, and compare it with the 6-5-4-3-2 nutrition countdown.

CHOOSING THE RIGHT GRAZING FOODS

Many of my clients have a difficult time figuring out what to eat for snacks. To make it simple, I have compiled a list of snacks for any occasion that you can keep in your office, home, backpack, suitcase, briefcase, or glove compartment. See figure 2.1.

If you are lucky and your office has a refrigerator, take advantage of it! Your options are increased when refrigeration is possible. Figure 2.2 suggests some possibilities. If you don't have access to refrigerator or if you are on the road a lot, consider using a portable cooler, especially the kind you can plug into your car's lighter. Also see chapter 6, "Meals at Work and On the Road." Table 2.1 lists brand-name snacks to give you a head start in stocking up your snack pantry. For more mini-meals ideas that take less than 60 seconds to fix, see chapter 13, "Creating 60-Second Specials."

To reap the benefits of grazing, there are a few key points to remember:

* Don't confuse eating more frequently with eating increased quantities of food. The benefits reported in grazing studies occurred when two groups of people on the *same number of calories* per day were compared; the only

The following snacks are especially handy to have on those days when you are racing against the clock. The foods listed here travel well.

Bagel	Energy bar
Bean soup in a cup (just add hot water)	Fig bars
Bran muffin	Half sandwich
Bread sticks, whole wheat	Juice box
Cereal, whole-grain	Mashed potatoes in a cup (just add hot water)
Cheese, low-fat, and crackers	Oatmeal in a cup (just add hot water)
Crackers, whole-grain	Raisin bread
Dried fruit	Tuna, snack-sized

Figure 2.1 Snacks to stash.

Many workplaces have refrigerators and even kitchens where you can store your food. These perishables make for nutritious grazing.

Applesauce, unsweetened	Salad
Cheese, low-fat	60-second meals (chapter 13)
Cottage cheese, low-fat or nonfat	Sliced chicken
Half sandwich	Sliced turkey breast
Leftovers	Yogurt, low-fat or nonfat

Figure 2.2 Chilling out: Snacks for the lunchroom fridge.

TABLE 2.1 BRAND-NAME SNACKS

Item	Serving size	Calories	Protein (g)	Carbohydrate (g)	Fiber (g)	Fat (g)	Saturated fat (g)	Sodium (mg)
Healthy Choice Microwave Popcorn	6 cups	100	4	22	5	2	0	330
Bumble Bee Fat-Free Tuna Salad*	1 can + 6 crackers	150	9	24	1	1.5	0.5	760
Fig Newtons	1 pkg	200	2	39	2	4	0.5	200
Nile Spice Couscous Minestrone Soup (soup in a cup)	1 container	180	8	34	2	1.5	0	590
Nile Spice Lentil Soup (soup in a cup)	1 container	170	0	34	11	1.5	0	540
Nile Spice Red Bean Soup (soup in a cup)	1 container	170	10	35	10	1	0	590
Nile Spice Split Pea Soup (soup in a cup)	1 container	200	13	35	8	1	0	600
The Spice Hunter Split Pea Soup (soup in a cup)	1 container	190	12	32	N/A	1	0	560
Pop Secret 94% Fat-Free Butter	6 cups, popped	110	4	26	4	2	0	380
Nature Valley Granola Bars (various flavors)	2 bars	180	4	29	2	6	0.5	160
Lean Pockets (Chef America)	128 g (1 piece)	270-290	10-13	38-48	2-4	7	2-3	470-790
Del Monte Fruit Cups	4 oz.	50-80	0	13-20	< 1	0	0	10
Del Monte Fruit Rageous	4 oz.	80-90	< 1	19-22	< 1	0	0	10
Del Monte Fruit To-Go	4 oz.	70-80	< 1	10	< 1	0	0	10

Item	Serving size	Calories	Protein (g)	Carbohydrate (g)	Fiber (g)	Fat (g)	Saturated fat (g)	Sodium (mg)
Cool Cut Carrots and Ranch Dip (Looney Toons)	2.25 oz.	60	1	6	< 1	4	0.5	200
Cool Cut Celery and Peanut Butter (Looney Toons)	2.25 oz.	170	5	9	< 2	14	2	30
Starkist Lunch-To-Go (Del Monte)	1 container	210	20	32	1.5	7*	1	720
Tree Top Fruit Rocketz (applesauce)	2.25 oz. (1 tube)	45	0	11	0	0	0	N/A
Quaker Oatmeal Express	1 container	200-210	4-5	41-42	3-4	2.5-3.5	0.5	250-320

* To reduce the fat, use half the mayonnaise.

difference was how the meals were divided up. The more eating occasions, the smaller the amount of food on each occasion.

▪ Be mindful of what you are eating. Mindless eating is a common pitfall that can lead to overeating.

▪ Choose foods using the 6-5-4-3-2 nutrition countdown. Grazing foods optimally should fill at least one of the food group servings that you still need that day. This helps to ensure that you get adequate nutrition from your snack. You may simply want to keep a running total in your head. You can keep track with the slash-tally method shown in figure 2.3. Or you can keep track on a sticky note in your appointment book or wherever it is convenient.

▪ Choose nutrient-dense foods. This means choosing foods that have the most nutrition for the mouthful in the least amount of calories. For example, a potato is considered nutrient dense compared with potato chips.

▪ Foods need to be portable and ready to go. Think how often you have made noble attempts to graze on vegetables, only to find them buried at

Grains	Fruits/ Vegs	Protein	Calcium-rich	Fish (weekly)
卌I	卌	IIII	III	II

Figure 2.3 Slash-tally method for tracking the nutrition countdown.

the bottom of the refrigerator, wilted. Solution: They should be washed and ready to grab or packaged and ready to eat, such as baby carrots.

▸ The food items need to be accessible. If you're working through lunch, your snacks need to be stashed in a briefcase or desk drawer.

FOOD FOR STRESS AND EMOTIONAL RELIEF

Many people do not feel comfortable about taking even a well-deserved break. They would never simply sit and relax at their desk "doing nothing" for a break because "it would look lazy." Consequently, to get a break many people turn to food, even when they are not hungry. Eating becomes a facade to look productive, an acceptable time-out.

Here is an example. Sally was a receptionist for a busy law firm and sought my advice for her "chocolate habit." After a few sessions it became quite clear that seeking chocolate was the only way Sally gave herself permission to take a break or just get up from her desk. Sally had no chocolate cravings at home. But at work Sally was required to remain at her desk at all times to greet all the incoming clients. The candy jar full of chocolate was located in the break room—a productive reason to get up from her desk. Sally's solution was to begin to take the two break periods to which she was entitled but for which she previously had trouble speaking up. Voila—the end of Sally's chocolate craving! I asked Sally what other alternatives she could come up with for taking a quick break. She was able to come up with several, now that she knew her true reason for heading to the lounge. Her alternatives included taking a quick walk outside, distributing mail, and getting up to ask her supervisor a question rather than e-mailing it.

Another statement I often hear from those on the quest to look and be productive is, "I get anxious if I suddenly have nothing to do." I find that people who are used to being productive and on the go feel very uncomfortable when a moment of "nothingness" unexpectedly occurs. It can come with an unexpected two minutes of free time, not enough time make a phone call or boot up the computer to check for e-mail. But foraging for food—whether a trip to the vending machine or the kitchen pantry—can often fill that void. If you have a tough time relaxing or unwinding, you might find yourself foraging when you get home after work or later in the evening. Ask yourself, Am I biologically hungry? If the answer is chronically no, you need to find nonfood solutions to fill the void, such as sinking into a comfortable chair and doing absolutely nothing or going for a brief walk.

Finally, there's the common element of *stress*. When the going gets tough, a lot of people turn to food, especially snacks. When 212 people were surveyed about stress and eating, 73 percent reported an increase in snacking. Although increased snacking doesn't automatically mean eating more, those who were the most vulnerable to overeating while snacking were dieters.

Energy Bars: Help or Hype?

One type of bar that can be beneficial is the energy bar. Energy bars are generally indestructible, which means that you can toss them into a suitcase, briefcase, backpack, or desk drawer for those unexpected times when you need a quick snack or bridge to your next meal. However, not all energy bars are created equal. Some have a surprising amount of artery-clogging saturated fat, while others offer very little fiber. When choosing a bar, be sure to read the Nutrition Facts label, or you could end up with a bar that more closely resembles a candy bar. Choose a bar that is low in saturated fat (less than three grams) and higher in fiber (at least three grams). When it comes to protein, many of the bars are loaded with more than you really need, especially when you factor in other foods that you'll eat during the day. The average man and woman need only 56 grams and 46 grams, respectively, of protein each day. Stick with moderate protein levels—around 10 grams is plenty. See table 2.2 for the nutrition profiles of some popular energy bars.

TABLE 2.2 ENERGY BARS

Item	Serving size (1 bar)	Calories	Protein (g)	Carbohy-drate (g)	Fiber (g)	Fat (g)	Satu-rated fat (g)	Sodium (mg)
Atkins Advantage Bar	60 g	220-250	17-21	2-3	7-11	8-13	4-8	65-200
Balance Bar	50 g	200	14-15	22-24	< 2	6	1.5-3.5	90-190
Balance Gold	50 g	200-210	15	22-23	< 1	6-7	4	80-125
Balance Oasis	48 g	170-190	8-9	25-29	< 1	1.5-3.5	1-2	220-270
Balance Outdoor	50 g	200	15	21	2-3	6	1-1.5	75-140
Balance Satisfac-tion	75 g	280	11-12	47-48	6	5-6	4	260-350
Balance+	50 g	190-200	14-15	22-23	< 1	6	3-4	80-160
Biochem Ultimate Lo Carb Bar	60 g	230-270	20-25	2	0	6-10	0.5-1.5	240-360

(continued)

TABLE 2.2 *(continued)*

Item	Serving size (1 bar)	Calories	Protein (g)	Carbohydrate (g)	Fiber (g)	Fat (g)	Saturated fat (g)	Sodium (mg)
Clif Bar Ice Series	68 g	250	10	43	5	5	1.5	120-140
Clif Bar Nutrition	68 g	220-240	8-12	39-44	5-6	2-5	0-2	135-290
Golean Bar (Kashi)	78 g	280-290	13-14	47-54	6-7	5-6	3-4.5	85-290
Layered PowerBar Protein-Plus	56 g	220	14-15	26-30	< 1	5-6	3.5-4.5	105-160
Luna Nutrition (Clif Bar)	48 g	170-180	10	24-29	1.5-2	2.5-4.5	0-3.5	120-190
Met-Rx	100 g	320-340	26-27	48-50	0-2	2.5-4	0.5-2	95-135
Met-Rx Protein Plus	85 g	290-310	31-34	25-32	1-2	4-9	1-7	75-160
Mojo Bar Nutrition (Clif Bar)	45 g	200	8-9	25-29	2	6-7	0.5-1	250-520
PowerBar Harvest	65 g	240	7	45	4	4-4.5	0.5-1	80
PowerBar Harvest Dipped	60 g	250	7	45	2-4	5	2	100-125
PowerBar Performance	1 bar	230-240	9-10	45	3	2-3.5	0.5	110
PowerBar Pria	65 g	110	5	16-17	N/A	3-3.5	2-2.5	70-80
PowerBar Protein-Plus	1 bar	270-290	24	36-38	1-2	5	2.5-3.5	140
Promax	75 g	280-290	20	35-44	0-2.5	4-6	2.5-4	140-220
Slim-Fast Breakfast and Lunch Bar	34 g	140-150	5	19-20	2	5-6	2.5-3	65-80

Item	Serving size (1 bar)	Calories	Protein (g)	Carbohydrate (g)	Fiber (g)	Fat (g)	Saturated fat (g)	Sodium (mg)
Slim-Fast Chewy Granola Bars	56 g	220	8	35	≤ 1	5-6	3.5	230-320
Slim-Fast Meal On-The-Go	56 g	220	8	33-37	2	5	3-3.5	100-160
Slim-Fast Nutritional Snack Bars	28 g	120-130	≤ 1	20-22	< 1	3.5-4	2-2.5	70-80
Sugar Free PowerBar Protein-Plus	48 g	170	16	19-20	1-2	4	2-2.5	110-135
Think Thin! Low Carb Bar	60 g	230-240	19-20	3	< 1	8-10	4-6	75-250
Think Thin! Protein Bar	65 g	270-280	22-23	18-19	< 1	9	4.5-6	210-240
Zone Perfect	50 g	190-210	14-16	20-24	0-1	6-7	1.5-4.5	190-360

ADVERTISING: SELLING THE SIZZLE

Many food companies exploit any iota of nutrition to make their foods sound redeeming. Fortunately, new food-labeling laws have closed many loopholes, but healthy-sounding descriptions on food labels may still give the illusion of wholesomeness, even when the opposite is true. Here are some examples to watch out for:

Healthy-sounding	*but*
Fruit rolls or bits	Often high in sugar
Juice drinks	Contain little juice
Granola bars	Often loaded with fat and sugar

Also beware of the commercial traps that lure you into believing that a candy bar (or the equivalent) is a nutritious treat to carry you over. Candy bars are usually packed with fat and sugar.

CHAPTER 3

Smart Shopping Strategies

Do you dread grocery shopping? I do. Ironically, I do enjoy spending time in the supermarket exploring new foods and labeling trends. In the haste to get grocery shopping over and done with, it's easy to unintentionally buy the wrong kinds of foods. Some convenience foods have an undeserved reputation for being healthy, and when you're too busy to read the label, you might be fooled by this halo effect. Sure, turkey is a very lean meat, but processed into bologna or a frankfurter, it's just another fatty food. Some foods just sound wholesome, like soup. But, Maruchan Instant Lunch (roast chicken flavor) is loaded with sodium, 1,380 milligrams (more than half of the recommended daily maximum intake), and the artery-clogging saturated fat is six grams (one third of the maximum recommended amount). Please keep in mind that no single food will ruin your health, but if you are consistently eating fatty or sodium-laden foods, a change may be in order.

SCANNING LABELS FOR NUTRITION FACTS

Thanks to the Nutrition Labeling and Education Act, it's possible to figure out what's in a food just by glancing at the Nutrition Facts section on a food label (figure 3.1). Nutrition Facts labels are on nearly every food in the grocery store. I give the condensed version, the core nutrition information with brief comments, in table 3.1.

Are you worried that this is too much to know while shopping? Don't worry—a shortcut is listed right on the Nutrition Facts label. It's the % Daily Value, or %DV, a quick way to size up the nutritional value of a food without resorting to memorizing maximum and minimum amounts in grams or carrying a calculator. The Daily Value number is a goal or target for the entire day. The Daily Value percentage indicates how close one serving of a particular food takes you to the goal. By the end of your day, you generally want to have eaten 100 percent or more of the Daily Value for fiber and nutrients such as calcium and iron. But for dietary culprits such as cholesterol, saturated fat, and sodium, be sure to eat no more than 100 percent of the Daily Value.

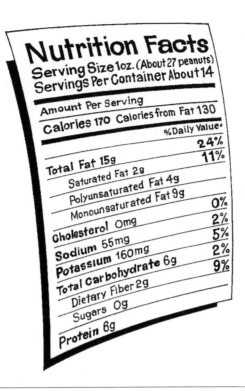

Figure 3.1 Nutrition Facts label.

TABLE 3.1 NUTRITION FACTS LABEL

Nutrition fact	Desirability	Comment
Calories	Not too many per serving	Be sure to check the serving size per package.
Total fat	The lower, the better	Maximum 65 g per day
Saturated fat	The lower, the better	Maximum 20 g per day
Cholesterol	The lower, the better	Maximum 300 mg per day
Protein	Generally desirable	The average person needs only 54 g per day.
Carbohydrate	Unless you are diabetic, not a key number to worry about	One average slice of bread has 15 g.
Fiber	More is better	The average person gets only half of what he or she needs daily. Aim for at least 25 g per day.
Sugars	Less is better	4 g is equivalent to 1 tsp. of sugar.
Sodium	Less is better	Maximum 2,400 mg per day

For instance, let's say you're trying to increase the fiber in your diet, and you are buying hot cereal. Cream of Wheat sounds high in fiber, until you look at the Daily Value. One serving provides only 4 percent of the Daily Value for fiber. There's nothing wrong with Cream of Wheat, but if you're looking for a fiber boost in the morning, you need to choose a cereal with a higher % Daily Value. For example, good old oatmeal provides 16 percent of the Daily Value for fiber for the day, a much better choice, but one that is not so obvious until you read the Nutrition Facts label.

Here are some other pointers for reading a food label:

Sugar

The USDA recommends limiting your sugar intake levels as follows:
    Maximum if you eat this number of calories daily:

6 tsp. (24 g)   1,600
12 tsp. (48 g)   2,200
18 tsp. (72 g)   2,800

Fiber

A high-fiber food has at least five grams of fiber per serving. Be sure to check the Daily Value for fiber (the higher, the better).

Fat

A low-fat food has three grams or less of fat per serving. Fat quality matters. Saturated fat is the type of fat that leads to clogged arteries and is required to be listed on the Nutrition Facts label. Another type of fat, *trans fatty acid*, is at least as harmful. Trans fatty acids may be even more damaging than saturated fats because not only do they raise the harmful blood LDL cholesterol, but they also lower the beneficial HDL cholesterol for a double whammy on the arteries.

Fortunately, a new law will require food companies to list the amount of trans fatty acids on the label; this takes effect in 2006. Until then, check out the ingredient label for trans fat sources—any food that contains hydrogenated oil contains trans fats (for example, margarine, baked goods, and fried foods). See table 3.2 for more insight on food label reading.

SPEED SHOPPING

Most of us consider grocery shopping an unpleasant chore: fighting the crowds, waiting in line at the checkout counter, unloading, and putting away our haul once we return home. Most of all, the whole process seems terribly time-consuming. Here are 10 timesaving tips to get you in and out of the grocery store quickly:

TABLE 3.2 FOOD LABEL LEXICON

Nutrient	What it means per serving
Calories Low calorie Reduced calorie	 40 calories or less At least 25% fewer calories
Cholesterol Low cholesterol Reduced cholesterol	 20 mg or less of cholesterol and 2 g or less of saturated fat At least 25% less cholesterol and 2 g or less of saturated fat
Fat Fat-free Low fat Reduced fat	 Less than 0.5 g 3 g or less At least 25% less fat
Fiber High fiber Good source of fiber	 5 g or more 2.5-4.9 g
Lean	Less than 10 g of total fat, 4.5 g or less of saturated fat, and 95 mg or less cholesterol
Extra lean	Less than 5 g of fat, 2 g or less of saturated fat, and 95 mg less cholesterol
Light	One-third fewer calories or 50% less fat
Saturated fat Low saturated fat Reduced saturated fat	 1 g or less of saturated fat and no more than 15% of calories from saturated fat At least 25% less saturated fat
Sodium Low sodium Light in sodium	 140 mg or less 50% less sodium
Sugar Sugar free No added sugar	 Less than 0.5 g No sugars, including ingredients that contain sugars such as juice or dry fruit, added during processing or packing

1. Use a list. Not only will it prevent another trip to the store for a forgotten item, but it's also faster.

2. Arrange your list according to aisle locations.

3. Avoid time-wasting aisles like the candy aisle.

4. Don't bother tasting samples. They are time wasters designed to tempt you to buy something that you don't want or need.

5. Bring only cash. It saves time at the checkout and prevents you from deviating from your list.

6. Divide and conquer. Divvy up the grocery list with a partner, such as your spouse, roommate, or kids.

7. Stock up on staples to cut down on trips.

8. Shop at a familiar store.

9. Shop during nonpeak hours. (Many stores are open 24 hours.)

10. Consolidate your buying at one store rather than several specialty shops if possible.

Quick Picks: Aisle by Aisle

There are over 49,000 items to choose from in a typical grocery store. How perplexing! The average number of products carried by a typical supermarket has tripled since 1980. Here are some pointers to help you choose the essentials, arranged by food categories.

Dairy Case

- Milk: Select nonfat, 1 percent, or 2 percent milk, including buttermilk.
- Cheese: Choose cheeses with less than five grams of fat per ounce.
- Yogurt: Choose nonfat or low-fat yogurts.
- Margarine: Buy the tub version with *liquid* oil as the first ingredient. (There's less trans fat in this form.) Go for the lowest-fat versions. If you must have the taste of butter, try the light butters, such as Challenge Light or Land O' Lakes Light; they have half the fat and calories of regular butter but still have a buttery taste.

Deli Case

- Lunch meats: Choose meats that have two grams of fat or less per serving.
- Hot dogs: Choose low-fat varieties; there are several.
- Fresh pasta: This is a quick-cooking alternative. But watch out for the filled pastas, such as ravioli; they may be high in fat.

Meat Case

Choose the leanest.

- Beef: The three leanest cuts are top round, eye of round, and round tip.
- Chicken: Buy skinless to save time (and fat), or buy with the skin and remove it yourself to save money.
- Pork: The tenderloin is the leanest part. Canadian bacon is leaner than traditional bacon.
- Turkey: Beware of processed cuts such as frankfurters, sausages, and bologna.

Breads and Cereals

- Bread: A whole grain should be the first ingredient, such as "whole wheat." The term "wheat flour" is merely white flour stripped of all its fiber. Check out the whole wheat pita bread, whole wheat flour tortillas, and whole wheat English muffins.
- Bread products: Beware of high-fat breads, such as croissants, pastries, doughnuts, biscuits, and scones.
- Cereals: Choose cereals with at least five grams of fiber.
- Crackers: Choose whole-grain, low-fat crackers. Beware of fatty crackers, such as Ritz crackers.

Canned Foods

- Beans: Stock up on a variety of beans (black beans, pinto beans, garbanzos, fat-free refried beans, and so forth). Even canned pork and beans is low in fat (only two to three grams of fat per serving).
- Fruit: Select those labeled "packed in own juice" or "no sugar added." Beware of "light" syrup; it has added sugar, although it is better than "heavy" syrup.
- Juice: Tomato or vegetable juice is a quick way to meet your vegetable quota. Make sure fruit juice is 100 percent juice rather than a sugary beverage with a hint of juice.
- Soups: Choose broth-based varieties, such as minestrone, chicken noodle, and vegetarian vegetable. Don't forget the bean soups, such as lentil, split pea, and navy bean. Soups can be a convenient way to get your vegetables in. Beware of cream soups, as they are high in fat.
- Produce: You can't go wrong here. Load up. Try the ready-to-eat, already-washed packages of salad, baby carrots, and chopped vegetables. Buy fruits in different stages of ripeness, so they are ready to eat when you are ready to eat them.

Freezer Case

- Frozen meals: Choose meals that have 800 milligrams or less of sodium and less fat, about three grams for each 100 calories. See table 3.3.
- Frozen breakfasts: Whole-grain frozen waffles, vegetarian sausages and links, and frozen bagels are good choices.
- Frozen produce: Pick frozen fruits, especially berries, and frozen vegetables such as spinach, peas, and broccoli.
- Desserts: Stick with 100 percent juice bars, sorbet, frozen yogurt, and lighter ice creams.

Miscellaneous

- Peanut butter: Choose brands without hydrogenated oil (which contains trans fatty acids). Try a natural-style brand, such as Laura Scudder's.
- Tuna: Buy water-packed.

Making the Most of Your Frozen Assets

Frozen meals can be great quick dinners. Just beware of these potential traps:

1. Most frozen dinners are not complete meals. They still require a little planning to ensure a day of balanced eating. This is especially true for entree-only meals that come with no side vegetables or accompaniments.

2. Beware of the salt mines! Many frozen meals are loaded in sodium. Keep in mind that the recommended sodium level for health is maximum 2,400 milligrams per day, which averages to a maximum of 800 milligrams per meal.

3. Frozen meals are typically lacking in calcium, vitamins A and C, and fiber. But you can easily make up for these deficits through grazing.

4. Keep in mind that the light meals, such as Weight Watchers and Lean Cuisine, are often more like a snack; they are actually too light in calories for some meals.

5. Hungry-Man meals (and similar brands) provide not only larger or extra portions but also a heap of extra, unwanted fat and sodium.

6. To round out your frozen meal with a nutrition boost, add one or more of the following: nonfat or 1 percent milk, raw or frozen vegetables, fresh fruit, a corn tortilla, a tossed salad, whole-grain bread, or whole-grain crackers.

7. Be adventurous: try the assorted frozen soy products. Stock up on veggie burgers. They are quick to make: just a couple of minutes in the microwave.

8. Watch the serving size. Many frozen pizzas appear to be "individual size" but actually contain three or more servings. For example, a California Pizza Kitchen BBQ Chicken Pizza provides three servings. Do the math: if you eat the whole pizza, that amounts to 840 calories, 27 grams of fat, and 2,100 milligrams of sodium.

9. Pot pies may sound healthy and complete because they contain vegetables, but they are usually loaded with fat calories.

TABLE 3.3 BEST BETS IN FROZEN CUISINE

Item	Serving size	Calories	Protein (g)	Carbohydrate (g)	Fiber (g)	Fat (g)	Saturated fat (g)	Sodium (mg)
Healthy Choice								
Bowl Creations	1 bowl	200-420	14-31	21-79	3-7	2.5-9	1.5-3	350-600
Choice Entrees	1 meal	200-350	9-25	19-46	2-7	3-9	0.5-3	520-600
Meals	1 meal	270-360	13-25	34-55	2-9	5-9	2-3	480-600
Meals To Go (Bread Stuffs, French Bread Pizza)	1 meal	310-360	17-22	46-58	1-8	5	1.5	590-600
Mixed Grills	1 meal	390-450	24-38	37-62	5-10	9-10	2-3.5	570-600
Lean Cuisine								
Café Classics	1 meal	290-370	16-20	36-54	3-5	2.5-8	1-4	830-890
Skillet Sensations	24 oz. (2.5-3.5 servings depending on size of portion)	180-250	8-15	23-37	1-4	2-9	0.5-2.5	430-630
Dinnertime Selections	1 meal	310-410	16-29	35-57	3-6	2-9	0.5-4.5	600-870
French Bread Pizza	1 meal	300-330	16-18	44-47	2-3	7-9	2.5-4	520-630
Weight Watchers								
Smart Ones Roast Turkey Medallions and Mushrooms in Sauce With Rice and Vegetables	240 g	213.6	15.1	34.6	3.1	1.7	0.4	504
Ultimate 200 Barbecue Glazed Chicken and Sauce With Mixed Vegetables	209 g	217.4	18.8	25.9	N/A	4.4	1	405.5
On-The-Go Chicken, Broccoli and Cheddar Pocket Sandwich	141 g	266.5	13.4	39.6	N/A	6.1	1.8	387.8

(continued)

TABLE 3.3 *(continued)*

Item	Serving size	Calories	Protein (g)	Carbohydrate (g)	Fiber (g)	Fat (g)	Saturated fat (g)	Sodium (mg)
Macaroni & Beef in Tomato Sauce	269 g	282.4	15.6	44.7	6.7	4.6	1.6	492.3
Chicken Enchilada Suiza, Sour Cream Sauce with Cheese	255 g	283	16.1	33.2	3.6	9.7	3.7	517.6
Smart Ones Lasagna Florentine	297 g	290	15	36	5	8	4.5	650
Smart Ones Bistro Selections Slow-Roasted Turkey Breast	10.0 oz.	220	18	20	2	7	2	660
Smart Ones Bistro Selections Peppercorn Filet of Beef	9.5 oz.	230	15	24	4	8	2	790
Smart Ones Santa Fe Style Rice and Beans	10.0 oz.	300	12	49	6	8	4	620
Smart Ones Tuna Noodle Gratin Made With Starkist Tuna	9.5 oz.	270	14	38	3	7	2.5	640
Smart Ones Spicy Penne Mediterranean	10.2 oz.	260	10	40	4	6	2	680
Smart Ones Bistro Selections BBQ-Style Chicken Pizza	7.5 oz.	400	19	65	3	7	3.5	730

PART II

Strategies for Dining Out

CHAPTER 4

Marvelous
Menu Choices

"I eat out every day at least two out of three meals."
—Sales representative

Once considered a luxury, eating out has evolved into a daily event, considered essential by many. Americans eat out an average of four times a week. Be it an occupational requirement or pure enjoyment, no other area of eating seems as challenging as eating out.

If you are not careful, eating out, especially on regular basis, can easily wreak havoc on your health. The average restaurant meal averages 1,000 to 2,000 calories and 50 to 100 grams of fat, according to Healthy Dining, a southern California company that has worked with restaurants since 1990 to help create and identify healthier menu selections.

The first step to healthy (but still tasty) dining is to "have it your way." Yet many people feel awkward making special requests. Remember that the restaurant business is a service industry that wants to meet your needs, especially in today's competitive market. It is only because of special requests that low-fat milk and low-fat salad dressing are now routinely available in restaurants. Specialty coffee shops even offer soy milk and soy lattes. These healthier choices have evolved because customers spoke up. Even if you are not able to get what you want this time around, you are paving the way for improvement by asking for it. I'll never forget ordering a pizza at a national restaurant chain and hearing the server ask if I wanted cheese on it! Clearly, this was a restaurant used to hearing and accommodating special requests.

Remember that you are the valued customer. You pay the bill and have the right to

- ask how the food is prepared,
- request that a food be fixed differently (such as broiled or without the sauce),

◢ send food back if it has not been prepared satisfactorily,

◢ ask for items not listed on the menu (such as grilled vegetables or lemon for your salad),

◢ request a doggie bag, even before the food is served,

◢ call the restaurant ahead of time to request that your food be prepared a special way (especially helpful if you have allergies, celiac disease [disease stemming from intolerance to gluten products], or other food intolerances),

◢ ask any question without fear of embarrassment or resentment from the server,

◢ leave if the restaurant cannot or does not wish to accommodate your needs, and

◢ expect special service because every customer is important.

STRATEGIES FOR EATING OUT

There are many ways to make healthy choices when eating out without feeling deprived. Keep these core guidelines in mind to ensure a healthier meal wherever you dine and no matter how frequently you eat out.

◢ Leave food on the plate. Combine the supersize servings offered by most restaurants with the clean-plate mentality and you have double trouble: more calories and fat than you need at one meal. Regardless of your size, restaurants serve you the same amount of food as everyone else. If you are in the habit of cleaning your plate when eating out, you are likely overeating, at least in the United States.

Breaking the clean-plate habit, especially when eating out, is one of the most important steps you can take. Even if you are dining out on a rich meal, if you leave part of the food behind, you take in only part of the calories. I find that most people truly understand the clean-plate trap and want to change, yet despite good intentions, they often wind up eating everything. The trick is to make eating a mindful event. Eating mindlessly, when you are not actually aware of what you are doing at the moment, makes it harder to change. Here are some techniques that can help.

• Put your napkin on the plate when you're finished; don't wait until your plate is empty. This signals the server that you have finished your meal, and your plate will be removed promptly if the service is good. Also, a napkin on your plate prevents unintentional nibbling if you linger over after-dinner conversation, as you are not likely to dig under the napkin for food.

• Place your fork and knife entirely over your plate, and be sure the handles are touching the remaining food. This too prevents mindless nibbling: no one wants to pick up a wet, soiled utensil.

• Request a doggie bag before the meal is served. Simply put half of your food in the bag when your meal arrives. Out of sight, out of mind.

To see the impact of cleaning your plate, check out table 4.1 for an idea of the amount of calories and fat you consume if you eat everything the restaurant serves you.

✎ Control where you eat. Whether you are eating alone or with a group of people, it usually takes a little time to decide where to eat, and where you eat can determine what you eat. Be prepared to name a couple of restaurants that have at least one healthy entree that you enjoy.

✎ Don't get caught in the get-your-money's-worth trap. Ever find yourself eating a lot of food to make sure you get a good deal? This can especially be a problem at buffets, salad bars, and brunches. Regardless of your economic background, there is something tempting about getting more than your money's worth when it comes to food. Many people also strongly value not wasting food.

Put more value on your health than on the quantity of food you consume. Consider the cost of coronary bypass surgery. It is no bargain if years of overeating lead to health problems.

✎ Never assume. Even though I am a registered dietitian, I am still surprised at the mistakes that I can make. Let me describe a few to save you from the same folly. In Boston, I once ordered what I thought would be a light meal: broiled scallops. Usually a broiled item is cooked dry. To my surprise, the scallops were broiled in butter. A few days later in New York, I ordered a shrimp salad with dressing on the side, expecting either jumbo or bay shrimp on a bed of lettuce. But I what I received was the equivalent

TABLE 4.1 CLEAN YOUR PLATE

Meal	Calories	Fat (g)
Prime rib dinner with Caesar salad and fully dressed baked potato	2,210	151
Seafood combo (fried fish with french fries, coleslaw, and 2 biscuits)	2,170	130
Lasagna with garlic bread and salad	1,538	77
Barbecue baby back ribs, french fries, and coleslaw	1,530	99
Chicken stir-fry with rice and egg rolls	1,213	62
Barbecue chicken sandwich (without fries)	1,072	46
Omelet with hash browns	850	53

Figures do not include beverage or dessert.

Source: Jones-Mueller et al. (2002), Jacobson and Hurley (2002), and www.dennys.com.

of tuna salad: chopped shrimp, heavy on the mayo. Never assume. Always ask how foods are prepared, even the basic items.

◢ Don't be afraid to make special requests. Get into the habit of having food served your way. Once, at lunch with a friend at one of my favorite Italian restaurants, she said, "I'm going to order your way." I don't tell my friends what to eat unless asked, so I was curious and a bit puzzled. She said, "I'm in the mood for salmon, but I want it on an entree salad." That's exactly what she ordered and exactly what she got—without opening the menu! Here are a few special requests to get you started:

- Low-fat or nonfat milk instead of cream for coffee
- Sauces and dressings on the side
- Whole-grain bread, especially for sandwiches
- Extra plate (to split an entree with a companion)
- Food grilled, dry broiled, or prepared with little oil
- Skin removed from chicken
- Fresh fruit or small green salad instead of french fries
- Hold the butter
- Baked potato instead of french fries
- Steamed or grilled vegetables without butter

◢ When you are famished, hold the bread or chips until the meal arrives. I can't tell you how many times my clients lament that they have a real problem

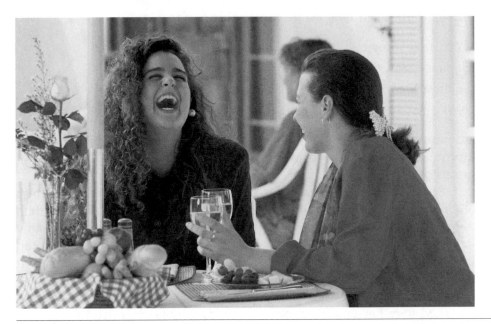

Eating out doesn't have to be tough: Select low-fat, low-sugar items and don't overdo the alcohol.

with eating too much bread. Bread is not the problem. It's hunger. When the server plunks down a basket of hot bread or chips, what's a famished person going to do while waiting for the meal to arrive? Eat it—and quite often, eat it all. The best thing to do in this situation is to ask that the bread or chips be served with the meal. You might be surprised what happens: you'll be more interested in eating your meal. The bread is not so irresistible when it does not have center stage, just equal billing with the entree.

 ▰ Pass on the bottomless refills for soda and other sweetened drinks. It's amazing how much soda can be refilled into your glass during your dining experience. Every 12 ounces gulped is another 140 calories. Three refills is 420 calories, just like that. Opt for brewed tea (iced or hot); not only is it calorie free, many studies show health benefits from drinking brewed black or green tea. Of course, water is always a terrific thirst quencher that's also easy on the budget.

 ▰ Check out the options labeled "healthy" on the menu. Thanks to restaurant nutrition labeling laws that went into effect in 1997, terms such as *light*, *low-fat*, and *healthy* have legal definitions. Menu items that are described with such terms are truly a better bet.

ORDERING HEALTHY

Believe it or not, you are not doomed to dull eating and you don't have to be a party pooper when you order a healthy meal. In some restaurants, it's only a matter of selecting an entree that already exists on the menu. For example, do these entrees sound tantalizing?

 ▰ Poblano turkey chili
 ▰ Steamed ginger sea bass
 ▰ Scampi Mediterranean
 ▰ Avocado swordfish with grilled vegetables

These mouthwatering dishes are examples of healthy entrees prepared by creative chefs from trendy restaurants. They are all under 350 calories and 15 grams of fat.

Just a few changes in your ordering style can make a big difference in calories without sacrificing fun and taste. Here's an example of how small changes made a big difference for my client, Don. Don had the pleasurable task of wining and dining his business's clients. However, Don's unlimited business dining budget brought with it the occupational hazard of weight gain. His meals usually began with a round of drinks and ended with dessert. Don wanted to lose weight while maintaining his professional duties. We worked together using a problem-solving approach, introducing only realistic changes that he was *willing* to make. The end result was a bit staggering: a savings of over 1,600 calories in one of his favorite restaurant meals. How was such a dramatic change made? Quite simply: by changing to one glass of wine rather than two cocktails, ordering a lighter appetizer and a lighter dessert, and changing the entree from a big steak to chicken. With consistent small changes, Don's weight dropped significantly, without going on a diet.

Figure 4.1, using nutritional data from Denny's restaurant menu, shows how making small changes adds up: saving from 499 to 688 calories at breakfast and from 1,339 to 1,721 calories at dinner! (Note that these calculations do not include beverage or bread basket.) If you eat out regularly, imagine what an impact a few improved choices can make.

DENNY'S BREAKFAST

Before

Item	Calories	Fat (g)
Original Grand Slam: two hotcakes, two eggs, two bacon strips, two sausage links	795	50
Maple syrup	143	0
Orange juice (8 oz.)	126	0
Coffee with 1 tbsp. cream	30	3
	1,094	53

Improved

Item	Calories	Fat (g)
Slim Slam: scrambled Egg Beaters, slice of grilled ham, and two buttermilk hotcakes	438	6
Sugar-free maple syrup	23	0
Orange juice (8 oz.)	126	0
Coffee with 1 tbsp. 2% milk	8	trace
	595	6

Lighter

Item	Calories	Fat (g)
Oatmeal	100	2
Cantaloupe	32	0
2 slices whole wheat toast, dry with jam	180	2
1 slice grilled ham	94	3
	406	7

(continued)

Figure 4.1 Revamping your ordering style.

DENNY'S DINNER

Before

Item	Calories	Fat (g)
Small Caesar salad with dressing	362	26
T-bone steak dinner with baked potato topped with 2 pats of butter and green beans	1,212	77
Hot fudge cake sundae	620	35
	2,194	138

Improved

Item	Calories	Fat (g)
Small garden salad with fat-free ranch dressing	138	4
Pot roast dinner with vegetable rice pilaf and green beans	437	16
Root beer float	280	10
	855	30

Best

Item	Calories	Fat (g)
Small garden salad with fat-free ranch dressing	138	4
Fit Fare: grilled chicken breast dinner with vegetable rice pilaf and green beans	275	9
Applesauce	60	0
	473	13

Figure 4.1   (continued).

AVOIDING MENU TRAPS

When you order a meal with your health in mind, it's disappointing to find out that your dinner is anything but healthy. Understanding restaurant menu jargon can help prevent that disheartening experience. Table 4.2 lists examples of menu jargon for both lower- and higher-fat dishes. Typical healthy-sounding menu items that may be just the opposite are given in table 4.3.

TABLE 4.2 MENU JARGON: HEALTHY OR HEAVY?	
Healthier Choice (lower in fat)	**Heavier Choice (higher in fat)**
Barbecued	A la king
Boiled	Alfredo
Broiled	Au gratin, cheese sauce
Charbroiled	Béarnaise
Grilled	Breaded or in batter
Healthy	Buttered, butter sauce
Heart-healthy, heart-smart	Cream sauce
In its own juice	Creamed
Low-fat	Crispy
Marinara	Fried, deep fried, pan fried
Marinated in juice or wine	Hollandaise
Poached	In its own gravy
Roasted	In puff pastry
Steamed	Marinated in oil or butter
Stir-fried	Meat sauce
Stuffed with vegetables	Melt, as in patty melt or tuna melt
Tomato sauce	Newburg
	Parmesan
	Scampi style
	Stuffed with cheese

DINING COURSE BY COURSE

Navigating your way through a menu can be tricky. This section highlights best bets and menu fare that is best limited, course by course.

Appetizers

Consider making a main course out of your appetizer. Often (but not always), the portion size is smaller. For example, try this appetizer meal: dinner salad, shrimp cocktail, and soup.

Best Bets

Fresh steamed vegetables, tomato juice, dinner salads, seafood cocktail, steamed or broiled seafood, nonfried egg rolls.

TABLE 4.3 HEALTHY-SOUNDING FAT TRAPS

Menu item	Problem
Breaded zucchini	Breaded usually means fried.
Buffalo wings	Whether baked or fried, this is chicken with the skin on.
Caesar salad	Salad dressing that clings to every lettuce leaf makes this a surprisingly fatty dish. Best to ask for either dressing on the side or less dressing when the salad is tossed.
Chef salad or Cobb salad	Usually loaded with dressing, cheese, eggs, and bacon, which can exceed the calories and fat in a cheeseburger. Hold the bacon and request the dressing on the side.
Quiche	Quiche is basically a savory pie with a cheese and cream filling. The crust alone is high in fat.
Salad bar	Surprised? If you stick with the raw fruits and vegetables, no problem. But creamy salads such as macaroni salad, potato salad, and pasta salad can be loaded with a lot of extra fat and calories. Accompaniments such as bacon, croutons, and dressing can easily make a salad add up to a 1,000-calorie meal (sans muffin).
Seafood platter	The fish is often fried. Best to ask how it's prepared.
Tuna salad sandwich	While tuna unadorned is certainly healthy, tuna salad glued together with mayonnaise is one of the fattiest sandwiches. According to the Center for Science in the Public Interest, the average restaurant or take-out tuna salad sandwich without extra mayonnaise on the bread has 720 calories and 43 g of fat. They should know: They purchased sandwiches from various shops and sent them to a lab for analysis.

Best Limited

Potato skins, fried vegetables (including onions), fried cheese, tortilla chips. A special note about tortilla chips: The biggest problem here is mindless munching. No matter how many times you push that chip basket away, your arm seems to find it. That magnetic phenomenon combined with the never-empty basket (thanks to a good server) usually results in your being full by the time the meal arrives. One solution is what I call the allocation method. Allocate about six chips to your bread plate (six because that is roughly equivalent to one tortilla). Have all the salsa you want, but savor those chips because when they are gone, adios. The difference is that an empty plate usually signals a stopping point, unlike the never-never land of the bottomless chip basket. Another solution is to request that the chips be served when the meal arrives.

Bread

If you arrive at a restaurant overly ravenous, it is best to request that the bread be served with the meal. If not, you may end up eating more than you intend out of sheer hunger.

Because bread is usually served hot and so is nice and moist, this is a good opportunity to cut down on butter or margarine. At restaurants that offer olive oil for bread dipping, keep in mind that while it is certainly a healthy type of fat, it has virtually the same number of calories as butter, teaspoon for teaspoon. If you can't do without a spread, use jam or honey.

Best Bets

Whole-grain bread, corn tortillas, flat breads, sourdough bread.

Best Limited

Croissants, muffins, biscuits, flour tortillas.

Salad

If you are not careful, your salad could easily drown in a bath of fat. A few dollops from an industrial-size dressing ladle can pack a big calorie wallop. A serving ladle holds about two ounces, or four tablespoons. The typical salad dressing has about 75 calories per tablespoon.

Best Bets

- Request dressing on the side, and spoon on your own dressing. Or try the "fork-dip-stab" method. Dip your fork into the dressing and then stab your lettuce. You get flavor in every bite but far fewer calories.
- When at a salad bar, put your dressing on the side in a soufflé cup or small paper cup.
- Explore the lower-fat salad dressings that are available at most restaurants.

Best Limited

Regular dressings, toppings such as bacon or crunchy chow mein noodles. Be careful with the cheese.

Soup

I consider a good soup a "speed-bump food," a food that inherently slows down the pace of your eating. It's difficult to eat hot soup quickly spoonful by spoonful.

Best Bets

Broth-based soups, such as vegetable, minestrone, or chicken noodle; bean-based soups, such as lentil, navy bean, or split pea.

Best Limited

Cream-based soups, such as cream of broccoli or cream of mushroom; cheesy soups, such as French onion or cheese and potato.

Entrée

Remember, never assume how an entree is prepared; always ask. Don't forget to inquire about the silent accompaniments that go with the entree, such as the vegetables and side dishes. Do make special requests that are suitable for you, such as these:

- Request an extra plate and split an entree with your dining partner.
- See figure 4.2 for specific best bets for international cuisines.
- Ask for a doggie bag in advance of the meal.

BEST BESTS IN ETHNIC CUISINE

Chinese

Appetizers/Accompaniments

Chicken wonton soup

Hot and sour soup

Sizzling rice soup (chicken or shrimp)

Spicy green beans

Steamed Peking ravioli

Steamed potstickers

Steamed rice, subgum soup

Steamed vegetable dumplings

Vegetarian delight

Velvet corn soup

Yu Hsiang eggplant

Entrees

Beef with broccoli

Chicken chop suey

Delights of three

Drunken chicken

Hunan tofu

Mandarin pancakes

Moo shu shrimp

Peking smoked chicken

Shrimp with broccoli

Shrimp with garlic sauce

Shrimp with tomato sauce

Sizzling sliced chicken

Stir-fried vegetables

Szechuan seafood

Teriyaki chicken or beef

Velvet chicken lo mein

Yu Hsiang chicken

Dessert

Lychee nuts

Cajun

Appetizers/ Accompaniments

Boiled crawfish

Boiled shrimp

Cajun rice

Candied yams

Cornbread

Fish sauce piquant

Oysters on the half shell

Smothered potatoes

Spicy tomatoes

Entrees

Baked fresh fish with crabmeat gravy

Crawfish boudin

Gumbo

Red beans and rice

Shrimp and crabmeat jambalaya

Shrimp and crabmeat spaghetti

Dessert

Lemon coffee cake

Figure 4.2 Try these best bets when ordering ethnic cuisine.

From *The Restaurant Companion* by H. Warshaw, 1990, Chicago, IL: Surrey Books (800-326-4430). Adapted by permission of the publisher. Also from *The International Cuisines Calorie Counter* by Densie Webb. Copyright 1990 by Densie Webb. Reprinted by permission of M. Evans & Co., Inc.

French

**Appetizers/
Accompaniments**

Baguette

Parsleyed ham in aspic

Puree of rice and turnips

Spinach braised with
onions

Vegetables melange

Entrees

Huitres fraiches

Scallop bouillabaisse

Steamed mussels

Veal stew

Desserts

Apples baked with rum

Apricot sherbet

Fruits frais et sorbet

Plums baked in custard

Raspberries (fresh) with
Chambord liqueur

Spice cake

Greek

**Appetizers/
Accompaniments**

Avgolemono

Baked beans, plaki style

Bean soup

Chicken rice soup

Chickpea soup

Green beans braised with
mint and potatoes

Lentil soup

Pita bread

Tomatoes and herbs with
rice

Tzatsiki

Entrees

Chicken souvlaki

Lamb with artichoke and
dill

Plaki fish

Shish kebab

Desserts

Carmel custard

Honey cheese pie

Japanese

**Appetizers/
Accompaniments**

Chicken and noodles in
miso soup

Chicken in grilled rice cake
soup

Clams and scallions in
bean soup

Miso soup

Peas and rice

Seafood sunomono

Shrimp in rice cake soup

Suimono

Su-udon

Sweet simmered Oriental
vegetables

White rice

Yaki-udon

Entrees

Glaze-grilled scallops

Nabemono

Pinecone squid

Pork and noodles in soy-
flavored broth

Sashimi

Shabu-shabu

Sukiyaki (chicken or beef)

Sushi

Teriyaki

Dessert

Fresh fruit

Indian

Appetizers/Accompaniments

Allu chat

Aloo chole

Biryani (shrimp or vegetable)

Chapati

Chickpeas and spinach mari-
nade

Chutney

Curried chickpeas

Dahl rasam

Kulcha

Lentils and spinach

Mulligatawny

Nan

Onion salad

Pulkas

Pullao (plain, with peas, or
with shrimp)

Rice pilaf with peas

Rice with chickpeas

Tamata salat

Tandori roti

Vegetable curry

Entrees

Bhuna (fish or lamb)

Chicken or fish tikka

Kheema matter

Lentils and vegetables with
chicken or fish masala

Rice and chicken pilaf

Saag (chicken or lamb)

Tandoori chicken or shrimp

Vindaloo (beef, chicken, or
fish)

Desserts

Fruit salad with thickened
milk

Mango

Pineapple fruit salad

Figure 4.2 *(continued).*

Italian

Appetizers/Accompaniments

Chickpea and pasta soup

Marinated calamari

Minestrone soup

Steamed clams

Entrees

Chicken cacciatore

Chicken marsala

Cioppino

Linguine with red or white clam sauce

Pasta marinara (without meat)

Shrimp marinara

Shrimp primavera

Spaghetti with eggplant

Stewed squid with tomatoes and peas

Veal cacciatore

Desserts

Fresh fruit whip

Italian ice

Rice cake

Mexican

Appetizers/Accompaniments

Black bean soup

Black beans

Ceviche

Corn tortillas

Gazpacho

"Pot beans" rather than refried beans

Salsa

Tortilla soup

Entrees

Arroz con pollo

Burrito (chicken, beef, or seafood)

Camarones de hacha

Fajitas (chicken, shrimp, or vegetarian)

Shrimp enchilada

Soft fish or chicken taco

Note: For combination plates, choose one entree rather than the "mucho grande" two or more entrees. Request vegetables in place of the rice.

Desserts

Capirotada

Flan

Middle Eastern

Appetizers/Accompaniments

Baba ghanoush

Couscous

Dolma

Ful medames

Hummus

Lentil soup

Miya dolma

Pita bread

Rice pilaf

Tabouli

Entrees

Kibbeh

Lah me june

Sheik el mashi

Shish kebab

Souvlaki

Dessert

Rice pudding

Thai

Appetizers/Accompaniments

Corn and shrimp soup

Crystal noodle

Pad jay

Papaya and shrimp salad

Pok taek

Seafood kabobs

Shrimp and orange chili salad

Squid salad

Steamed mussels

Steamed rice

Sweet and sour cucumber

Talay thong

Tom yum koong

Vegetable boat

Entrees

Garlic shrimp

Poy sian

Seafood platter

Scallops bamboo

Sweet and sour chicken

Thai chicken

Desserts

Lychee nuts

Mangoes and sticky rice

Thai fried banana

Figure 4.2 (continued).

Best Bets

Grilled fish, grilled chicken. If you are craving red meat, pot roast and sirloin steak are the leaner options.

Best Limited

Cheese-based entrees, fried foods, large meat portions, pot pies, meatloaf, and quiches.

Sandwiches

Contrary to popular belief, it's not the bread that can be problematic with sandwiches—it's the filling and how it's fixed. Even a lean-meat sandwich can be trouble if it's swimming in mayo and regular cheese. A tuna salad sandwich best illustrates this dilemma. Although tuna is naturally lean, once mayonnaise is added, tuna salad becomes of one of the highest-calorie sandwich choices on the menu.

Best Bets

Roast beef, turkey breast, grilled chicken, grilled fish. The best-dressed sandwiches use mustard or barbecue sauce rather than mayonnaise. Request light mayonnaise, or ask that mayonnaise be used on only one slice of the bread. Be careful with vegetarian sandwiches; some are loaded with cheese and mayonnaise.

Best Limited

"Salad" sandwiches, such as tuna salad, chicken salad, and egg salad; cheesy sandwiches, such as tuna melts and patty melts. Hold the bacon. If you crave a sandwich of this type, order the popular half-sandwich combo, which is usually a half sandwich with either soup or salad.

Beverages

It is very easy to guzzle calories, especially in this era of bottomless refills. When it comes to alcoholic beverages, it's best to keep it simple, such as a glass of wine rather than a cocktail, and it is better to order wine by the glass. If you order by the bottle, it's easier to drink more than one glass.

Best Bets

Mineral water, brewed tea (iced or hot), nonfat milk.

Best Limited

Regular sodas, milk shakes, lemonade.

Dessert Tray

Desserts once in a while are not a problem, especially if you get in the habit of sharing dessert or just savoring a few bites. Unfortunately, desserts too are growing in size. Remember when a piece of cheesecake was a thin sliver because it's so rich? Now it's cut to the size of a brick!

Best Bets

One dessert and many forks. It's surprising how just a couple of bites of dessert can be very satisfying, especially after a good meal. Or finish your meal with a coffee drink, such as a fat-free latte or fat-free cappuccino. Other good dessert choices include sorbets (especially homemade ones), fresh berries (without cream), chocolate-covered strawberries, and frozen yogurt.

Breakfast

Ordering breakfast might seem challenging because of fewer options, but it need not be. I once ate breakfast with a reporter who was very curious to see what I would order. I chose pancakes (no butter) and orange juice. The reporter was surprised that I did not hold the syrup and that I do not recommend that practice. Why? Food needs to taste good! I know very few people who enjoy eating dry pancakes. Or course, I am not suggesting that you drown your hotcakes in syrup. When available, fresh fruits, such as berries or bananas, are healthy breakfast toppings.

Best Bets

Omelettes made with egg substitutes or egg whites, pancakes, fresh fruit platter, cold or hot cereal, lox and bagels (easy on the cream cheese, or make it light cream cheese), whole wheat toast, fruit juice, tomato juice, and vegetable juice. Hold the butter or margarine; it is often served by the scoop. Jam or honey is a better choice than butter for a bread spread.

Best Limited

Biscuits, gravy, croissants, regular omelets, the 2-2-2 type of meal (two eggs, two sausages, two pancakes, two strips of bacon, too much fat). If you must have a breakfast meat, Canadian bacon, or even ham is an improvement over sausage or bacon.

Buffets and Salad Bars

Remember, your personal challenge is not to get more than your money's worth but to enjoy a healthy and tasty meal. Begin with a healthy mind-set. Consider brunches and buffets as simply a visual menu. You don't order everything on the menu even if every item looks good, right? Similarly, you are not obligated to try everything on the buffet.

Best Bets

Use a two-tiered approach. This strategy requires making two trips (an appealing thought). On the first trip, help yourself to the fresh fruits and vegetables and broth-based soups. This high-fiber start provides bulk to take the edge off your hunger, and you'll be in better control of your food choices when you come back for trip number two. To avoid the food-piling phenomenon, get in the habit of taking taste-size portions. Remember that the serving utensils are industrial size, and it's easy to inadvertently wind up with a plate piled high as Mount Everest. When you start eating, make sure the foods you eat are "taste bud worthy": don't finish the foods that don't taste good. If you don't love it, don't bother.

Best Limited

- Overflowing champagne. After one round, have the server remove your glass, or you may drink more than you want.

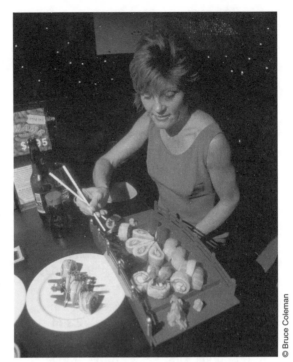

If you're thinking of a buffet dinner, try something more nutritional like a sushi bar.

- Goopy salads and casseroles. More often than not, the goop that holds these foods together is fat, so go easy on these items.

- Desserts. Desserts. Desserts. These tantalizing goodies are usually the first item you face at a brunch, yet how often have you bitten into a rich-looking chocolate cake only to discover that it's not what you expected, not so moist or not so chocolatey. Finishing a less than fabulous dessert is truly a waste of calories! If you are dining with a group of people, share one dessert plate of samples.

Rid yourself of the clean-plate mentality. If you don't like it, don't eat it. At a buffet, you probably cannot take advantage of a doggie bag. (Otherwise, some people would abuse the courtesy and bag a couple of meals.) The reality is that some food will go to waste. But remember, better wasted than *waisted!* Figure 4.3 shows clear cut examples how making better menu choices really add up in saving the calories and cutting the fat.

Day	Instead of	Try	The Difference a Choice Makes in:			
			Calories	Fat (g)	Saturated Fat(g)	Sodium (mg)
1	California Pizza Kitchen BBQ Chicken frozen pizza (whole)*	Wolfgang Puck's frozen Vegetable Primavera Pizza (whole 10.8 oz)*	240	1	7	900
2	Marie Calendar's frozen Chicken Broccoli Pot Pie**	Healthy Choice Honey Glazed Chicken frozen dinner	780	64	20	1180
3	McDonald's M&M McFlurry	McDonald's Hot Fudge Sundae	280	10	5	90
4	Baja Fresh Steak Nachos	Baja Fresh Taco Steak Combo Meal (2 soft tacos, beans)	1611	96	0	0
5	Burger King Fries, King size, salted	Burger King Fries, Small size, salted	370	19	5	660
6	Denny's BBQ Chicken Sandwich w/o Fries	Denny's Fit Fare Grilled Chicken Breast Dinner	642	39	8	1507
7	32 ounce regular soda	32 ounce iced tea, unsweetened, + 1 sugar packet	314	0	0	11
	One Week Savings		4237	229	45	4348

How These Changes Stack Up, Line-by-Line

	Calories	Fat	Saturated Fat (g)	Sodium
California Pizza Kitchen BBQ Chicken	840	27	14	2100
Wolfgang Puck Primavera Pizza	600	26	7	1200
Difference	240	1	7	900

Figure 4.3 Eating on the Run Modification Chart.

	Calories	Fat	Saturated Fat (g)	Sodium
Marie Calendar's Chicken Broccoli Pot Pie	1100	70	22	1760
Healthy Choice Honey Glazed Chicken Dinner (chicken, vegetables & roasted potatoes)	320	6	2	580
Difference	780	64	20	1180
McDonald's M&M McFlurry	620	22	14	260
McDonald's Hot Fudge Sundae	340	12	9	170
Difference	280	10	5	90
Baja Fresh Steak Nachos	1958	102	N/A	N/A
Baja Fresh Taco Steak Combo Meal (2 soft tacos, beans)	347	6	N/A	N/A
Difference	1,611	96	N/A	N/A
Burger King Fries, King size, salted	600	30	8	1070
Burger King Fries, Small size, salted	230	11	3	410
Difference	370	19	5	660
Denny's BBQ Chicken Sandwich w/o Fries or fries substitute	1072	46	10	2309
Denny's Fit Fare Grilled Chicken Breast Dinner w/glazed carrots and baked potato	430	7	2	802
Difference	642	39	8	1507
32 ounce soda (no ice)	378	0	0	20
32 ounce iced tea (no ice), 1 packet sugar	32	0	0	9
Difference	314	0	0	11

*While the stated serving size is for more than one portion, most people I counsel eat the entire "salad-plate size" pizza. Data is for entire pizza.

**While the stated serving size is two portions, most people I counsel eat the entire pot pie (which looks like one serving). Data is for entire pot pie, which is also comparable to what's served in a restaurant for one person.

Figure 4.3 *(continued).*

CHAPTER 5

Fast Food Without the Fat

"I really don't like to eat fast food, but because of my daughter's gymnastics lessons, my son's soccer, my husband's meetings, and my full-time work schedule, it's often the best we can do for dinner."—Marketing manager

It's no secret that fast-food places are not the bastion of healthy eating. But you *can* eat at a fast-food place and fare relatively well. Almost every fast-food establishment has at least one healthy (or healthier) choice. But first, let's look at the potential problems if you enter the arena of fast food mindlessly.

When you are in the "gulp-and-go" cycle, you may not give a second thought to what you put into your body. I find that even my health-conscious clients tend to fall into the all-or-none trap the moment they enter a fast-food restaurant. They rationalize, "Since I'm eating fast food, I might as well blow it." This mind-set combined with the ease of ordering combo meals and their inexpensive supersizing can quickly spell trouble. Even if you are not supersizing, some foods by themselves exceed a day's worth of fat and sodium if you eat the whole thing. Table 5.1 gives a few examples.

TABLE 5.1 FAST FOOD FACTS

	Calories	Fat (g)	Saturated fat (g)	Sodium (mg)
Baja Fresh Chicken Nachos	1,920	102	N/A	N/A
Burger King Original Double Whopper with cheese	1,150	76	30	1,530
Del Taco Macho Beef Burrito	1,170	62	29	2,190
Hardee's Monster Burger	1,060	79	29	1,860
Jack in the Box Ultimate Cheeseburger	1,120	75	28	2,260

If you want to see how your favorite fast-food order stacks up nutritionally, check out appendix A, "Fast-Food Nutritional Charts." You'll find nutrition information on 22 fast-food companies, including pizza places, sandwich shops, and take-out places.

Now let's focus on the positive, that is, how to make the best out of a fast-food situation. Keep in mind that in a pinch, fast food can be better than going too long without eating, which can lead to overeating.

Here are some guidelines to help make the best of your fast-food order.

* Don't assume that because a menu item sounds healthy, it is. While a chicken sandwich sounds healthy (and it can be), if it's fried or loaded with bacon and cheese, it can be much higher in fat than a hamburger, which is particularly sad if that's what you wanted all along! For example, Arby's Market Fresh Roast Chicken Sandwich has 820 calories and 2,160 milligrams of sodium, more than one day's maximum recommended sodium.

* Forget supersizing. While it's tempting to get more food for mere pennies, in the long run you may pay a bigger price with your health.

* Opt for charbroiled or roasted sandwiches, especially chicken.

* Hold the mayo. Try using mustard or ketchup instead, or request light mayo, available at many places.

* Consider quenching your thirst with low-fat milk, orange juice, or iced tea.

* Have a sweet tooth? Take advantage of the frozen yogurt offered at many fast-food places.

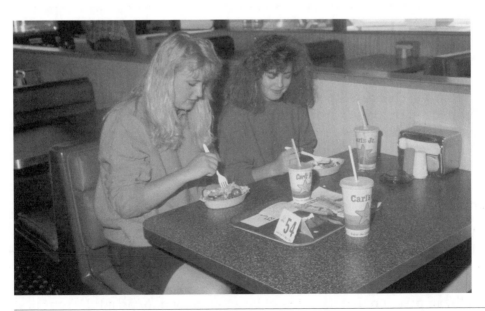

Anytime you eat fast food, beware of money-saving tricks like "super-sizing."

Want Fries With That?

Once you navigate around the main entree, the inevitable question will be asked: "Do you want fries with that?" In the old days, you could order small fries; you'd get about 200 extra calories, which, although not the healthiest, is not really a problem once in a while. Today many fast-food places no longer offer small fries except with the kid's meal and instead offer assorted extra large sizes. These supersized behemoths rival the calories of a McDonald's Quarter Pounder With Cheese, as you can see in the following table!

BATTLE OF THE BULGING FRIES

	Calories	Fat (g)
McDonald's Quarter Pounder With Cheese	530	30
Arby's Large Homestyle Fries	560	24
Burger King King Fries	600	30
Carl's Jr. Large Fries	620	29
Del Taco Macho Fries	690	46
Hardee's Monster Fries	510	24
Jack in the Box Super Scoop Fries	580	28
McDonald's Super Size Fries	610	29
Wendy's Great Biggie Fries	530	23

 • Opt for entree salads or side salads, but go easy on the dressing. Better yet, request the light salad dressing.

 • Gotta have the fries? Then choose the smallest size.

 • Hold the cheese. Although cheese is rich in calcium, it is loaded with saturated fat. Until the fast-food industry offers lower-fat cheeses, save your cheese eating for home or grazing times when low-fat varieties are available.

 • Limit anything fried. This includes the healthy-sounding alternatives chicken and fish. Once these items are fried, they are not healthier choices.

What if you are in the mood for a burger? A basic small burger is really not so bad, and it can be a good source of iron, a mineral that most women and children do not get enough of. The problem is getting a basic burger, which in most fast-food places has been relegated to the children's menu, giving you the impression that it could not be enough food for an adult. Your best bet is to request a small hamburger and round it out with a side salad (most places have them) with light dressing. If you are also in the mood for fries, order the kid's meal; you'll get a small burger and small fries.

Homestyle Take-Out

A general rule of thumb is that anywhere you can get a vegetable with a meal, you can end up with a decent meal. This is especially true of homestyle take-out places such as Koo Koo Roo and Boston Market. Entrees range from grilled chicken or turkey replete with many healthy side options, such as steamed vegetables, baked beans, and corn on the cob. While there are fantastic options here, you can't assume that every dish is dandy in the nutrition department. For example, an open-faced turkey sandwich at Boston Market will give you 720 calories and over a day's worth of sodium (2,850 milligrams), while a hand carved turkey dinner at Koo Koo Roo racks up 881 calories and 4,229 milligrams of sodium.

Deli Do's

In sandwich shops, the six-inch (or small) size is a better bet, regardless of what's in it, than the foot-long size. No rocket science here: it doubles everything. Of all the sandwich shops, Subway deserves an honorable mention for promoting an array of healthier sandwiches that are low in fat. (They've also benefited nicely, as sales are up 40 percent since introducing this promotion of healthier sandwiches in the mid-1990s.) Follow these tips to keep your sandwiches healthier:

- Choose whole wheat bread; it's an option that adds a nice fiber boost to lunch.
- Request extra lettuce, tomatoes, onion, and bell peppers. It's an opportunity to get vegetables in.
- Choosing the leanest cuts of meat can make a tremendous difference. Lean meats include roast beef, turkey, and chicken.
- Beware of the healthy-sounding tuna salad and chicken salad sandwiches. They are among the fattiest choices on the menu due to the mayonnaise both in the salad and on the bread.

Pizza

Pizza can be a nutritious choice and a great source of calcium if you stick with just a couple of slices. Depending on the pizza maker, two slices of a medium pizza provide 25 to 40 percent of your calcium needs for the day. Best bets include cheese or veggie pizza on a thin or hand-tossed crust.

While individual pizzas are convenient for one person, they can rival the nutritional profile of one McDonald's Quarter Pounder With Cheese. For example, a Pizza Hut cheese Personal Pan Pizza has 630 calories and 28 grams of fat. Compare that with a Quarter Pounder With Cheese at 530 calories and 30 grams of fat. Part of the problem is that individual pizzas tend to be deep-dish style, hence higher in calories and fat. Deep-dish pizzas are often dripping with oil to help slide the pizza out of the pan. If you are dining alone, you are generally better off ordering two individual slices of a thin-crust cheese or veggie pizza. Round out your pizza meal with a side salad.

Smoothie Shops

As long as you consider a smoothie more of meal than a snack, for the most part you will be fine. Generally, smoothies provide about 400 to 500 calories. Be sure to choose smoothies that contain whole fruit and, optimally, yogurt rather than sherbet or ice cream. Some smoothie shops offer a free nutritional add-on, such as vitamins, protein, or fiber. Most smoothies are low in protein, so it is best to opt for the protein boost. The fiber content should already be adequate if you choose whole-fruit smoothies.

CHAPTER **6**

Meals at Work and On the Road

"I travel all the time; it's hard for me to eat right."
—CEO of a national company

Power meals and cutting deals, meetings drowning in doughnuts, and logging frequent-flier miles are examples of occupational eating hazards. This chapter gives some quick tips for navigating around tricky eating conditions that can be found in any job.

AT WORK

The easiest way to keep business casual is to eat. Often the most important deals are made as you wine and dine potential clients, hashing out details over filet mignons and shaking hands over lime sorbet. When it comes to business, any business, time is the key factor, and time is something no one has enough of. The following sections give some tips on surviving the business eating routine, eating well without losing the deal.

Morning Meetings and the Coffee Routine

My motto is "Breakfast—don't leave home without it." Breakfast needn't be a big meal; a light morning snack helps keep you from being vulnerable to poor eating decisions. On an empty stomach, anything goes, including an unintended doughnut during a morning meeting. It's one thing to eat that doughnut if you really want it, but eating out of hungry desperation feels quite different and often results in eating more food.

Overdoing the coffee is also a problem. Many people drink coffee at meetings to fight boredom. If it turns into an all-day meeting, that's quite a load of caffeine. Slowly sipping one cup (eight ounces) of coffee an hour can easily result in drinking 8 to 10 cups a day. Keep in mind that if you use a coffee mug, you are likely drinking 12 ounces, or a cup and a half, of coffee each time you empty the mug. Following are some strategies for curbing the coffee habit.

- Be sure to arrive at meetings with breakfast or snack in your stomach. If possible, find out in advance who orders the food for the meetings, and request that fresh fruit, bagels, and yogurt be included in the menu.
- Limit coffee to two cups (16 ounces) a day.
- For a good night's sleep, finish coffee drinking by noon.
- Consider switching to decaffeinated coffee.
- Your best bet is to use nonfat milk rather than cream.

Business Meals and Cutting Deals

The goal of power meals is not power eating but rather accomplishing your agenda, be it creating new business or networking. This is all the more reason to keep your food simple and healthy. Who wants spaghetti on their face or spinach dangling on their teeth when trying to make an impression? Focus your energies on the conversation, not on what you are eating. This isn't the time to indulge in a meal that you are not likely to savor. How could you possibly savor your meal when your mind is focused on your business objective? So here's a good strategy:

- Stick with simple, easy-to-eat foods.
- Order a lighter meal, such as grilled chicken or grilled fish.
- Stick to your healthy restaurant requests (see chapter 4 if you need ideas).

Vending Machine Roulette

Many of us have played the game of vending machine roulette. It's late afternoon, your stomach starts to growl, and you turn to the vending machines. These are some of the best choices from the vending machine:

- Pretzels
- Fruit
- Mini-box of cereal
- Chocolate milk
- Sunflower seeds
- Peanuts

If these choices are not available, ask the person responsible for stocking the vending machine if they can be included, or bring your own snack. Be careful of eating as a way to escape afternoon monotony.

Catering Trucks

Many people call these traveling food establishments "roach coaches" but, in spite of this, continue to frequent them. The familiar horn blows, and workers flock to these at-your-door food venues. The challenge here is that most foods are already prepared and wrapped to go; catering trucks are like movable vending machines. If you are a regular customer, make your requests for the next day so that they can be fulfilled at the master kitchen. For example, request that a turkey sandwich be prepared only with mustard and no mayonnaise. Your best bets include nonfat yogurt, bagels, juice, and nonfat or low-fat milk.

Unpredictable Schedules and Eating Interruptus

Thanks to cell phones and beepers, the end to a well-planned schedule is only a beep or ring away. You are often at the mercy of the caller. Physicians, fire fighters, on-call workers, and others who may be needed at a moment's notice in a crisis are especially vulnerable. Sales representatives, quality assurance people, and managers also are often called away to solve problems. Such interruptions may make eating seem impossible. If you have an unpredictable schedule, try these strategies to get you through the day.

- Keep a stash of grazing snacks in your work environment (review chapter 2).
- Take advantage of the office kitchen if you have one; keep it stocked.
- Remember not to go longer than five hours without eating.

OFFICE POLITICS: EATING YOUR WAY UP THE CORPORATE LADDER

You may be working very hard to impress your superiors with your corporate work ethic in order to climb your way to the top. If so, consider eating necessary for the survival of the corporate fittest. How can you do your best work when you are running on empty? Beware of the following pitfalls at the office.

Working long hours. Putting in long hours at work, whether by choice or demand, can do you in nutritionally if you are not prepared. It is all too easy to go longer than five hours without eating if, for example, you eat lunch at noon and don't get off until six or when you are so bombarded with work that you literally don't have time to think about food. On days when you know you will put in extra hours, plan ahead and stock your desk, briefcase, or company refrigerator with energizing grazing snacks or pack a double lunch. During unexpected late hours, take a food break. If time is so precious that you can't even make it to a fast-food place (see chapter 5 for healthy choices), have the food delivered. Not only does food fuel your brain cells, a food break can enhance productivity by allowing you to "unplug" for just a bit.

Eating in the executive dining room. Eating in the executive dining room is not only a perk but an opportunity to network with key people in the corporation. Unfortunately, executive dining is not immune from unhealthy food. If possible, ask the chef to prepare your foods without the customary butter and sauces. If your company has an on-site wellness program, suggest the dining service work with it by offering at least one healthy entree. Eating-out strategies from chapter 4 also work here.

Office potlucks and birthday parties. Nothing beats the lunch-box blues like an office potluck or birthday party, but these events cause a lot of eating pressure. I'm not sure which is more challenging, a well-meaning relative trying to cajole you into eating a certain food or a coworker coercing you to "try it." Consider bringing something delicious that just happens to be healthy. I'm always pleasantly surprised at how quickly fruit plates or veggie plates get devoured. When filling your plate, use the same strategy as for buffet dining: begin by taking taste-size portions. If you want to partake of the birthday cake or dessert, be sure to savor it. And if it tastes mediocre or disappointing, toss it.

Food gifts. "Thank you," says an appreciative client and sends you a tin of cookies. "Job well done," says a boss and gives you a box of chocolates. Obviously, you do not want to return their appreciation with ingratitude. Fortunately, the solution is easy: share the wealth. An occasional treat is not a health disaster for you or your colleagues, but don't pressure your colleagues into eating something they don't want either. A local food bank will accept any food offering.

Desktop goody jars. Goody jars often invite people into your work space, which can be fun but also a nuisance or an unwanted distraction. If you are prone to mindless eating, your desktop is not the best spot for a treat jar. Keep food off your desk to help discourage mindless eating.

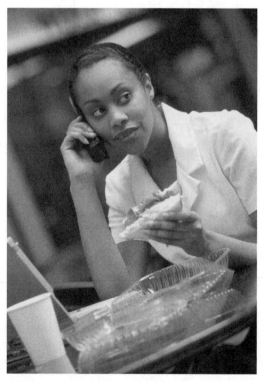

Food is fuel for your brain. You need food to keep you at your best.

◢ **Giving at the office.** Girl Scout cookies, Little League candy bars . . . it seems as if one colleague or another is always helping their kids out by selling goodies as a fund-raiser. Give a donation if you feel inclined, but since the purpose of selling the treats is to raise money, giving money without ordering the goods is not in bad taste.

◢ **Happy hour.** An after-work get-together can be a fun way to get to know colleagues in a relaxed atmosphere. But alcoholic beverages and accompanying appetizers can be a meal (or more) in themselves. Try ordering mineral water with a twist. Remember that the purpose of happy hour is to network and socialize with coworkers. If you drink alcohol, stick with simpler beverages such as wine rather than cocktails. Best bets for appetizers include nuts, popcorn, mini-tacos, pretzels, oysters, shrimp, and crab.

ON THE ROAD

If your job requires travel by car or plane, you have many healthy food options wherever your job takes you. You might just need to be more creative in some situations. In this section, we look at how to handle road trips and travel.

At the Hotel

To keep fit while on the road, seek hotels that have gym facilities and bring a set of workout clothes. Pack a pair of walking shoes; walking is a great way to get to know a new city or just get fresh air. Ask the concierge or front desk if they have course maps for walking or running, and find out where the safest areas for walking are. Check out these national hotel chains to see if they have facilities at your destination with a gym or with healthy entrees on their restaurant or room service menu.

Hotel	Web site	Phone number
Doubletree	www.doubletree.com	800-222-8733
Embassy Suites	www.embassysuites.com	800-362-2779
Four Seasons	www.fourseasons.com	800-332-3442
Hyatt	www.hyatt.com	800-233-1234
Holiday Inn	www.holiday-inn.com	800-465-4329
Hilton	www.hilton.com	800-445-8667
Radisson	www.radisson.com	800-333-3333
Ritz-Carlton	www.ritzcarlton.com	800-241-3333
Sheraton (Starwood)	www.sheraton.com	800-325-3535
Marriott	www.marriott.com	800-228-9290

In the Car

Sales reps, truckers, reporters, and others who spend time on the road daily are subject to eating pitfalls. Fast food quickly gets boring, and time to actually sit in a restaurant is a rare luxury. Some people opt for a shorter lunch to wind up the day. One of the most clever solutions I've heard was from a local television news cameraman who is constantly racing to the next newsmaking scene. He installed a microwave in his news van so that he can heat up nice meals no matter where he is!

Another strategy is to keep a portable cooler stocked with easy grazing snacks and beverages. Electric coolers that plug into the cigarette lighter offer the convenience of not needing ice, but you need to keep the cooler plugged in. Be sure to keep cash on hand for when you need to eat—whether it's a healthy fast-food option, a smoothie, or a latte.

At the Airport

Logging frequent-flier miles doesn't mean an end to your healthy diet. But sometimes long trips or unexpected delays can make you vulnerable to both jet lag and meal drag. There's nothing worse than being stranded at an airport with the food stands closed while dinner is flying high without you. A delayed plane can mean a delayed or missed meal.

When the food court is open, you may find familiar foods with recognizable names that can be quite appealing while waiting for your plane. Eating in airports is similar to eating out, so the restaurant tips discussed in chapter 4 apply here as well. Fortunately, airport cuisine has improved considerably, with many healthful options for you to choose. A 2002 survey of the 10 busiest U.S. airports by Physicians Committee for Responsible Medicine (PCRM) found that healthy meal options abound (at some airports more than others). Table 6.1 gives PCRM's airport food ratings. The physicians' group reviewed food establishments for at least one entrée that met these

Killing Time Without Food

For some weary travelers, eating might seem to be the most exciting thing to do in the airport. If this sounds like you, you could be headed for distress by using food to beat boredom. Familiar names such as Mrs. Fields or Fannie May may seem especially comforting in a strange city. Your best bet is to plan ahead. Bring along extra reading material or even some work to do. Some airports offer amenities such as on-site health clubs and barber or beauty shops. Take advantage of them. The best extra two hours I ever spent in an airport were in Dallas, where I indulged myself with a massage and manicure. That's what I call effective stress relief!

**TABLE 6.1 PCRM'S AIRPORT FOOD RATINGS 2002:
AVAILABILITY OF HEALTHY FOOD CHOICES AT THE 10
BUSIEST AIRPORTS IN THE COUNTRY**

Airport	Score	Healthy restaurants/Total restaurants
San Francisco	96%	25/26
Denver	79%	26/33
Los Angeles	54%	32/59
Dallas	53%	33/62
Houston	50%	16/32
Atlanta	49%	25/51
Phoenix	48%	19/40
Las Vegas	45%	20/44
Minneapolis	44%	20/45
Chicago	42%	25/59

A restaurant was rated healthy if it offered at least one low-fat, high-fiber, cholesterol-free entree. The percentage score is the number of healthy restaurants divided by the total number of restaurants.

The Airport Food Rating Survey is available at www.pcrm.org/news/health021113report.html

criteria: low fat, high fiber, and cholesterol free. San Francisco International Airport landed an impressive mark: 96 percent of all its restaurants offer a healthy option. This survey did not include yogurt and coffee shops if they did not offer an entrée, nor did it rate as healthy foods with any cholesterol, which means a negative rating for otherwise healthy options such chicken or fish. Therefore, the number of healthy entrees available is likely higher than indicated. Here is a sampling of airport cuisine that met the criteria: portobello mushroom sandwich, sushi, veggie burrito, vegetable stir-fry, bean burrito, and veggie burger.

On the Plane

One of the best tips I received for airline meals was from a seasoned commercial pilot. His advice was to order the special meals. Ironically, his reason was not health; he found the taste to be consistently superior. I have also found the special meals to be very tasty. The types of special meals available vary considerably, depending on the airline carrier, but they tend to fall into three classes:

- **Religious:** Kosher, Hindu, Moslem
- **Special diet:** Diabetic, low-cholesterol, low-sodium, vegetarian
- **Other:** Light, bland, seafood platter, child's

In most cases, ordering a special meal is simply a phone call away. You can do it when you make airline reservations. Most airlines require 12 to 24 hours' notice. You can't beat the price of special meals: no extra charge. See table 6.2 for the special meals offered by several major airlines.

TABLE 6.2 AIRLINE SPECIAL MEALS

	Alaska Airlines	America West Airlines	American Airlines	Continental Airlines	Delta Air Lines	United Airlines	US Airways
Hours of advance notice needed	24	12 (24 for kosher)	24	24	12	24	24
Type of meal							
Baby food/ infant				X	X	X	X
Bland	X		X		X		X
Child's	X			X	X	X	X
Diabetic	X	X	X	X	X	X	X
Fruit plate	X			X	X	X	X
Gluten free			X	X	X		X
Heart healthy			X				
High fibers						X	
Hindi				X	X	X	X
Islamic			X	X	X	X	X
Kosher	X	X	X	X	X	X	X
Lactose free or low				X			
Low calorie	X	X	X	X	X	X	
Low calorie and low cholesterol							X
Low cholesterol		X	X				
Low fat							X
Low fat and low cholesterol	X			X	X	X	
Low protein						X	
Low purine						X	
Low sodium	X	X	X	X	X	X	X
Obento Japanese						X	

	Alaska Airlines	America West Airlines	American Airlines	Continental Airlines	Delta Air Lines	United Airlines	US Airways
Peanut free							X
Seafood				X	X		X
Soft			X				
Vegan						X	
Vegetarian	X	X	X		X		X
Vegetarian, Asian				X	X	X	X
Vegetarian, lacto-ovo			X		X	X	X
Vegetarian, nondairy			X				

Here are some tips to keep you well-nourished on your journey.

- Get in the habit of reserving a special meal when you make your plane reservations.
- When ordering a special meal, ask the agent for an explanation of the meal. Not all special meals are created equal; they vary from airline to airline.
- When you board, let the flight attendant know that you have ordered a special meal. That way, if the airline forgot to load your special meal, the flight attendant may be able to correct the oversight before takeoff.
- If your special meal does not arrive, ask for a meal voucher.
- Bring some standby snacks, just in case. Snacks that travel well include nuts, dried fruit, and energy bars.
- Drink one cup of water for every hour in flight to minimize dehydration.
- If you don't a have special meal, avoid adding fat such as margarine.
- For breakfast, opt for the cold cereal, which usually comes with fresh fruit and low-fat or nonfat milk.
- If you are scheduled for a lunch or dinner meeting when your plane arrives, request either a *special* fruit plate or a light snack to avoid double meals.
- Be sure to check your itinerary for meal service. Never assume that a meal will be served.
- No time to order a special meal? Reserve your seat toward the front of the plane; you are more likely to have a choice of all meals offered before one runs out.

- If you are traveling first class, be sure to make special requests when ordering from the first-class menu. For example, ask that your salad dressing be served on the side.

PART III

Solutions for Everyday Living

CHAPTER **7**

Losing and Maintaining Weight

"Diets are only second to sex in popularity among discussions in my office."—Los Angeles talk show host

So many otherwise intelligent and successful people nevertheless succumb to the latest diet fad because they want the pounds off yesterday. Combine desperate people with questionable (at best) diet books or the latest info-mercial weight-loss program and you have the latest top-selling weight-loss fad. To illustrate this desperation to lose weight, in the year before fen-phen was pulled from the market, about 18 million people took this prescription weight-loss medication.

Yet we do have another sad trend in this country: more adults and children are obese than ever before. Nearly 65 percent of adults are overweight or obese, yet in 1980 only 15 percent of adults were obese. The overweight rate for children and adolescents 6 to 17 years old has doubled to 10 to 15 percent. If dieting truly worked, then why is this weight-gaining trend escalating?

WHY DIETING FAILS

Quick diets usually just put your lifestyle on hold temporarily. You don't learn how to deal with challenges such as eating out, eating in social set-tings, eating while traveling, or stress eating. Instead, you merely postpone dealing with these situations.

You may indeed lose weight, but not for long. When the diet is over, you are likely to revert to your real lifestyle and easily regain the weight. Even worse, the weight regained may make your body fatter, even if you go back to your old weight before dieting. This is because crash diets promote water and lean-tissue (muscle) loss. When you inevitably gain the weight back, you don't gain back the muscle you lost; you gain fat. Your body has a vital need for energy in the form of carbohydrates. If you are not getting enough carbs or energy from what you are eating, your body cannibalizes muscle. It breaks down the protein from muscle into amino acids, which in turn are converted to glucose to supply energy to the body, especially the brain. Muscle is 75 percent water. So when muscle tissue breaks down, water is released. Two cups of water weigh one pound. If a program promises that you will lose 10 pounds in one week, ask yourself, 10 pounds of *what?* To lose 10 pounds of fat in one week, you need an energy deficit of 5,000 calories a day!

The Life Span of a Diet

Study after study has shown that the more you diet, the harder it becomes to lose weight. Your body becomes more resistant to dieting. It seems that the body can tolerate only a certain number of dieting assaults; then it revolts. When you go on a crash diet, your body thinks you are starving it. It doesn't know that the lack of food is only temporary. As a result, it adapts by going into starvation mode and conserving every calorie you give it. Your metabolic rate slows down, which lowers your caloric requirement, making it even easier to regain the lost pounds. Consider the results of these two studies: One study of 112 overweight women found that the most successful in losing weight had the lowest number of repeated dieting attempts. Another recent study of over 10,000 boys and girls, ages 9 to 14 years, found that frequent dieters are significantly more likely to become overweight than those who never dieted, regardless of their intake of calories or their physical activity level.

Consequences of Dieting

Repeated dieting has more than just metabolic consequences. A study of 350 dieters and nondieters found that dieting impairs memory. The volunteers were given tests of memory, reaction time, and mental processing capacity. Lead researcher Mike Green, of the Institute of Food Research outside London, found that the mental deficit triggered by dieting was similar to that seen in someone who just had a lot to drink! Interestingly, those who ate a little less food for health reasons but were not dieting had no mental impairment.

Dieting can also slow reaction time according to the research of Molly Kretsch of the Western Human Nutrition Research Center. Fourteen female volunteers went on a strict reducing diet for 21 weeks. During that period, reaction time slowed by 11 percent and continued to slow for three weeks after the dieting was over. Imagine trying to slam on the brakes of your car with this reduced reaction time!

Dieting affects your mind and mood. The more you diet and the more severe the diet, the more likely you are to obsess and worry about food. It's not unusual to experience increased irritability and mood swings. Also, failed attempts at weight loss through dieting often bring self-hatred and guilt. But it's the diet that has failed you, not you who have failed at dieting.

Unfortunately, for some, dieting is the springboard to an eating disorder. According to the National Eating Disorders Association, 35 percent of so-called normal dieters progress to pathological dieting. Of those, 20 to 25 percent progress to partial or full-blown eating disorders.

Convenience and Liquid Diets

While programs such as Jenny Craig and Nutri/System say they incorporate behavioral education and sound nutritional habits, there are problems with such plans. A major problem is that while you are eating packaged diet food, you are not living in the real food world, making decisions about what to eat and so forth. For example, business people have told me that they would pull out their diet food packets in a restaurant while their clients dined on regular menu fare. This behavior does not last long because it is not realistic and it ignores the core issue of how to order in a restaurant without doing in your health or waistline.

Diet programs may discuss these issues or lecture on behavior change, but all the while you are on some canned or packaged diet. This does not seem effective. It's like trying to learn how to play the guitar by hearing someone describe how to do it without the benefit of actually playing or struggling to reach a chord with your own fingers. Liquid diets, such as Slim-Fast, that replace one or two meals seem easy but ignore the real eating problems. Some people attest, "All it took to lose weight for good was Nutri/System (or Slim-Fast)." I wish them well, but the odds are just not good with these approaches.

High-Protein Diets

There has been a lot of hype about high-protein diets but very little research, let alone long-term studies. Let's face it, anyone can lose weight temporarily; maintaining the weight loss is problematic. The American Heart Association in a science advisory statement advised against high-protein, low-carbohydrate diets for these reasons:

1. High-protein diets may increase uric acid levels and trigger gout in susceptible people.
2. These diets may raise blood pressure because they limit fruits, vegetables, and nonfat dairy products. These foods are rich in potassium, calcium, and magnesium, which have a beneficial effect on blood pressure.
3. High protein triggers loss of calcium in the urine; this obviously is not good for bone health. Most Americans don't get enough calcium in their diets as it is.

4. High-protein diets eliminate or limit the foods that decrease cancer risk.

5. High-protein diets that are also very low in carbohydrates provide only one fifth of the carbohydrates necessary to prevent loss of lean muscle tissue.

6. People on high-protein diets may find it difficult to complete exercise or may easily become exhausted when exercising as a result of both low carbohydrate intake and inadequate glycogen stores. (Glycogen is the storage form of carbohydrate. Muscle glycogen provides energy exclusively to exercising muscles.)

There are also other problems with high-protein diets. A recent study demonstrated that high-protein diets can cause serious dehydration in athletes. When the body metabolizes protein, one of the by-products, urea, is excreted through the kidneys, which requires the excretion of extra water as well.

Another problem with high-protein diets is that they may interfere with your brain's neurochemistry. Making the "feel-good" chemical, serotonin, requires the amino acid tryptophan in the brain. Tryptophan is easily acquired from protein-rich foods such as turkey. Yet to get tryptophan from the food you eat into the brain (where all the serotonin construction takes place), it needs to cross the blood-brain barrier. Carbohydrate is required for this to happen, because it triggers the release of insulin, which then enables tryptophan to cross through the blood-brain barrier. But high-protein diets are typically low or very low in carbohydrates.

To make this even more complicated, eating a lot of protein (which breaks down into amino acids) interferes with tryptophan's crossing into the brain through a competitive inhibition process. It's like trying to get a taxi in New York on a rainy day; it's much harder to get a ride because tryptophan is competing with the extra amino acids.

A recent study by Reidel and colleagues demonstrated that when people were depleted of tryptophan (by drinking a special protein solution), half of those with a family history of depression reported feeling blue. And 9 percent of volunteers with no family history of depression had a decline in mood. Memory was also impaired.

Finally, some very low carbohydrates diets claim that triggering the body into ketosis (making and using ketones) rather than using carbohydrates as a fuel is safe. Ketones are an alternative fuel source used by the body when the diet is too low in carbohydrates. But research shows that the heart loses contractile function when using ketones as fuel. (Although this is finding was from rat studies, it is compelling.) Ketones eventually need to be excreted from the body via urine. But this results in loss of the minerals calcium, magnesium, and potassium.

Dieting Fads

If you are trying lose weight quickly scrapping one diet only to go on another is a waste of time and could damage your metabolism. The biggest time waster is cycling through losing and gaining the same pounds over and over again by dieting. You can save time by steering clear of fad diets. Here are some tips to avoid becoming a notch on the belt of the latest futile approach to fat loss.

- If it sounds too good to be true, it probably is. Sorry, you can't dream or melt your weight off, no matter what the infomercials say.
- If it promises fast weight loss, you will probably be losing the wrong kind of weight: water and muscle. Remember that two cups of water weigh one pound; quick weight loss usually means lost water and muscle.
- A complete program should include at least a combination of exercise, lifestyle management, and a nutritionally sound program that is flexible, not rigid. For example, does the program
  - allow you to eat out and give guidance on how?
  - accommodate your eating style, whether it's grazing or meal-based?
  - consider social situations?
  - promote realistic eating? For example, if you don't like to cook but suddenly you are required to cook extravagant dishes with exotic ingredients, you could be in for problems.
  - include a cognitive behavioral element? Cognitive behaviorism looks at how your thoughts affect how you feel, which in turn affects how you behave (in this case, eat). For example, if you thought that by eating one cookie you blew it, and this caused you to feel guilty and ineffective, you might behave by eating several more cookies. Yet if you were to readjust your thoughts by saying, "Eating one cookie is normal; it's not going make or break my health," you might feel okay and accepting and behave by eating just the one cookie.

What About Fat?

Keep in mind that our bodies require two essential fats, linoleic acid and alpha-linolenic acid, just as we require vitamins. One group of fats in particular, the omega-3 fatty acids (of which alpha-linolenic acid is one) have additional health properties, from lowering triglycerides to improving mood.

When it comes to fat, most Americans get more than they need (except for the omega-3 fatty acids). Fat has twice the calories of any other energy nutrient, so it makes sense to cut some of the excess here, where you won't miss it. For example, a tuna salad sandwich from a restaurant often has mayonnaise in the tuna mixture *and* on the bread. Best to have the tuna without the added mayo on the bread: you won't even miss it. Similar changes can easily be made in your favorite recipes.

Try substituting lower-fat options in your favorite recipes. You're likely to continue eating lower-fat versions of your favorite foods if you experiment and keep an open mind.

Try serving a leaner version of a food to guests or family members, but don't tell them about it until after they have tasted it to avoid prematurely biasing their taste buds. Don't forget that small changes make a big difference, especially if repeated consistently over time.

1. Try at least two low-fat substitutions (see table 7.1).

2. Remove excess fat. Skim fat off meat juices when making gravy. Drain fat from browned meat. Remove skin from chicken.

3. Try low-fat cooking techniques: steam, broil, poach, grill, or roast, and use nonstick sprays or nonstick pans.

4. Love the taste of butter? Try light butter, which tastes great but has half the fat and calories.

5. Check food labels, and choose the lower-fat option if the food is comparable in the taste-bud department.

TABLE 7.1 ALTERNATIVES TO HELP LOWER FAT

Instead of	Substitute	Calories saved
Dairy		
1 cup whole milk	1 cup nonfat milk	70
1 cup heavy cream	1 cup evaporated skim milk	621
1 cup sour cream	1 cup fat-free sour cream	244
	1 cup nonfat plain yogurt	621
1 cup cheddar cheese	1 cup low-fat cheddar cheese	120
8 oz. cream cheese	8 oz. light cream cheese	200
	8 oz. fat-free cream cheese	586
	4 oz. light cream cheese + 4 oz. fat-free cream cheese	394

(continued)

What About Fat? *(continued)*

Instead of	Substitute	Calories saved
Fats		
1/2 cup oil	1/2 cup applesauce	907
	1/4 cup applesauce + 1/4 cup oil	454
1 stick margarine or butter	1/2 cup applesauce	747
	1/2 cup light margarine	400
2 tbsp. oil	2 tbsp. wine or broth	159
1 cup cream soup	1 cup evaporated skim milk + 1 tbsp. flour + 1 bouillon cube	149
Proteins		
2 whole eggs	4 egg whites	94
1 lb. regular ground beef	1 lb. ground turkey breast	839
	1 lb. ground turkey	358
	1 lb. extra lean ground beef	123
	1 lb. diced chicken breast	585
6 1/2 oz. tuna in oil	6 1/2 oz. tuna in water	182
Miscellaneous		
1 cup chocolate chips	1/2 cup mini chocolate chips	251
1 cup shredded coconut	1/2 cup shredded coconut	233
	1 tsp. coconut extract	337

WEIGHT MANAGEMENT ON THE RUN

It's important to begin with a good mind-set. Here are two keys.

1. Progress, not perfection. This positive mind-set will get you through tough times and help you maintain perspective. Remember that minor eating indiscretions will not affect your health or weight—it's what you eat routinely. Believing that you must be perfect in your eating habits can send you into a downward spiral that results in throwing in the towel. What's important is to learn from your eating experience and move on.

2. No forbidden foods. Surprised? Here's why. If I told you, "Do not think of a pink elephant," what would pop into your mind? A pink elephant! Likewise, if you are not "allowed" to eat ice cream, cake, or cookies, all you can think about are these forbidden foods. One of my clients told me that her favorite part of a diet was going off it. She would plan for weeks the foods in which she would overindulge.

The restraint theory explains this all-or-none eating phenomenon. Studies have shown that people who are very rigid and restrained about what foods they eat tend to overeat when a disinhibitor comes along. A disinhibitor can be any event or situation that causes a person to give in to a forbidden food. Giving in may happen for the following reasons:

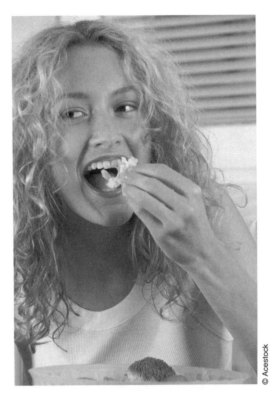

Eating well as often and consistently as you can will help you on the road to a long and healthy life.

- A person may feel the urge to indulge *now* because the diet begins again on Monday (as usual), and this may be the last opportunity ever to have this food. This can cause people to eat as though it were the "Last Supper," to get it while they can.

- A person who cannot eat forbidden food without rationalizing or feeling guilty has never truly enjoyed the food but rather eats it fast, as if to deny even eating it or to hurry up and get on with the guilt.

- A person who has felt deprived for a long time may not trust his or her ability to handle a forbidden food and overeats after one bite.

The point of not forbidding any foods is to learn how to have a satisfying experience with food without overeating. For example, five scoops of ice cream don't taste any better than one or two; chances are that your taste buds are frozen by the time you're down to the last few scoops. Keep in mind that having a healthy relationship with food is just as important as healthful eating. *Intuitive Eating*, which I teamed up with Elyse Resch to write, describes this important process in much more depth.

Taking Action

Let's look at some quick but effective strategies to start achieving a healthful weight for your body. Here are four basic steps to help you with challenging areas:

Step 1. Identify problem areas by keeping a food journal. Be sure to include a weekend. Keep in mind that this is just a tool to discover key eating habits and triggers. This is not a tool to beat yourself up with! Here are some items to note in your journal:

- Location where you ate (kitchen, office, bedroom, and so forth)
- Duration (how long it took you to eat)
- Mood (for example, bored, stressed, angry, lonely)
- Simultaneous activity (watching TV, reading, surfing the Internet, and so forth)
- Did you clean your plate?

What are your eating trends? Your journal may reveal that you wolf down your meals in 10 minutes even when you are *not* racing against the clock. Or you may notice that when you feel stressed out, you find your hands in a box of cookies. Perhaps you tend to eat nonstop once you arrive home from work or school.

Step 2. Identify the priority areas that you would like to change. Then look over the following six action strategies and decide which can most affect your eating.

Step 3. Make changes gradually, for example, only one or two changes per week. If you try to do everything at once, you may feel frustrated and overwhelmed. It's best not to move on to changes in another area until you feel your new habits are established.

Step 4. Monitor your progress. Monitoring can be as simple as writing an accomplishment on a piece of notebook paper, such as, "I left food on the plate rather than cleaning it at the restaurant." It's easy to forget the changes you make or to take them for granted if you don't document them. I see this happen all the time!

Triggering Your Appetite

Different situations can trigger eating. For some people it might be emotional hunger. For example, stress, boredom, or anger triggers some people to eat. For others, grocery shopping on an empty stomach causes impulse buying of goodies. Recognizing your eating triggers can help you cope with those situations, events, or emotions without needing to turn to food. Once you have identified your key food triggers, it is time to take action. Following are some strategies that may help.

Emotions   Emotional eating does not necessarily mean that you are undergoing intense feelings such as stress, anger, or loneliness. In fact, little voids can be significant eating triggers for people who are used to being busy and multitasking. The moment they experience an unexpected moment of down time, food urges suddenly come up, and they turn to the vending machine or lunch room. Try these strategies:

- Identify your feelings. If you have difficulty doing this, many people find that the description "uncomfortable" often fits.

- Making a *realistic* list of activities to cope with your emotions. These activities should ideally be incompatible with eating. For example, to combat stress, get a massage, get a manicure, listen to your favorite soothing music, or close your eyes and try some deep breathing. Keep the list on hand. I find that a simple three-by-five-inch note card works pretty well, as it fits almost anywhere.

Social Pressure and Parties   The pressure to nibble at parties and other social gatherings can be intense. Instead of piling your plate full (and incidentally finding your mouth and hands too full to visit or shake hands), try these strategies for eating with etiquette.

- Mentally practice ways to decline offers of food that you really don't want.
- Eat a small snack before going to a party.
- Mentally plan how much alcohol you will drink.
- Stretch out alcoholic beverages by adding lots of ice (if appropriate) or a no-calorie mixer such as mineral water.

Grocery Shopping and Impulse Eating   How many times have you run in to the grocery store just for something for supper and come out with a whole cartful of goodies? This happens more times than most of us care to admit. Instead of those impulse buys, try these ideas.

- Try carrying just enough cash for planned purchases, as this will reduce impulse buying.
- Shop from a list.
- Shop when you are *not* hungry.
- Plan your snacks.
- Go no longer than five hours without eating.
- Plan your meals.

Cooking, Serving, and Storing Food   We all know it's hard to resist just one more bite, especially when there isn't quite enough to put away but too much for a whole second serving. Instead of feeling obligated to empty each dish, try these suggestions:

- Keep the serving dishes off the table (leave them in the kitchen) to prevent nibbling when you are not hungry.
- Put leftovers away immediately.
- Beware of unconscious nibbling while preparing food.
- Try using a small taster spoon rather than a cooking spoon when sampling a dish.

Changing the Act of Eating

Changing just one or two ways that you eat can often significantly reduce your intake without making you feel deprived. You may have heard of some of the action ideas in this section before, but have you ever tried to do them consistently? Any plan for change takes consistency and repetition. For example, you cannot realistically expect to build muscles by doing one push-up, deciding that it doesn't work for you, and brushing it aside. The same goes for making changes in your eating.

Unfortunately, life in the fast lane often breeds fast eating techniques that can be hard to change. Just because your life is fast-paced does not mean that *every* meal has to be gulped down in no time flat. On the days when you have a little extra time to sit and eat a meal, try these strategies; you will find that eating is more satisfying. Some of these strategies lengthen the duration of a meal. Keep in mind that it takes about 20 minutes for your brain to realize that your stomach is full. If you habitually eat faster than that, it's much easier to overeat.

➤ **Beginning of the meal.** When possible, do not engage in activity when you are eating. While this sounds simple enough, this activity is quite difficult for chronically multitasking people. If you don't focus your attention on eating, you may not notice that your meal is now inside you, and you may not feel that you've eaten. In *Breaking Free From Compulsive Eating*, Geneen Roth describes this situation as "the sense of being somewhere but not really being there, the 'sorry, how's that again?' feeling. The conversation or event took place, but because our attention wasn't present, it didn't take place for us, in us." Try designating only one spot for eating (such as the dining room or kitchen). This will help you become a conscious eater.

➤ **During the meal.** Swallow completely before beginning your next bite of food. Don't use a beverage to help swallow the food more quickly. Savor the flavors: How does the food taste? Does it taste as good as you imagined? What about the texture and temperature of the food?

➤ **Ending the meal.** Rate your hunger level from 1 to 10 *before* you eat (1 being painfully ravenous, 5 comfortable, and 10 painfully full). Try to stop eating when you feel that you are at 6 rather than continuing until the plate is empty. This exercise takes practice. You can also prevent unintentional eating by putting your napkin on your plate when finished or putting your eating utensils over the plate when finished (you are not likely to pick up goopy utensils to nibble).

EXERCISING

One key step to maintaining a healthy weight is routine physical activity. In fact, the 2002 report on Dietary Reference Intakes for energy and macronutrients recommended engaging in 60 minutes of daily moderately intense physical activity to prevent weight gain and to reap the other health benefits of exercise. (Be sure to check with your physician before beginning any exercise program.)

1. Start slow and simple. If the idea of exercise is overwhelming, begin just by moving your body. For example, if you sit at a computer all day long, your brain might be racing like an Olympian, but your body has had no movement. Movement can be as simple as walking around the office for 10 minutes. Try moving your body for at least 30 minutes a day; it does not have to be all at once.

2. Choose an activity that is fun for you, whether it's hiking, dancing, or riding a stationary bike while reading your favorite book.

3. Fit activity into your work style, and try putting it in your appointment book so that it becomes a nonnegotiable priority. Consider these times for working out:
   • During lunch
   • During breaks
   • After work

4. When traveling, stay at hotels that have gyms, or at least a stationary bike. Pack a jump rope. Bring walking shoes (a great way to tour a city). Check the local TV listings for a fitness show.

If you need support, try exercising with a friend or hire a certified personal trainer. And remember to think positive! As Henry Ford once said, "Believe you can or believe you can't. Either way you will be right." Your attitude can greatly affect how you behave and feel.

1. Dwell on your progress, not your shortcomings.
2. View any setbacks as a learning experience.
3. Set realistic goals.
4. Remember: progress, not perfection.

CHAPTER 8

Eating for Health and Longevity

"I was so busy, I didn't care about what I ate—until I found out that my cholesterol was off the chart."—Attorney

What you eat can play a big role in preventing many chronic diseases, such as heart disease, diabetes, and cancer. Yet as you speed full steam ahead into your schedule, you may be eating too much of the dietary culprits associated with these diseases or too little of protective foods and nutrients. Are you too busy for nutrition? While most people agree that their health is important, healthier eating often gets postponed until "I have time," "after I finish the project," and so on. If you do not have time to be sick, it's especially important to make the time to stay well! Make sure your food foundation is a solid one that can reduce your chances of disease.

Two landmark scientific reports that were years in the making—the 1988 *Surgeon General's Report on Nutrition and Health* and the 1989 Diet and Health Report both clearly show that nutrition can make a difference in preventing chronic diseases. And the recently released two-volume tome by the Food and Nutrition Board of the Institute of Medicine published in 2002, *Reference Intakes for Energy, Carbohydrates, Fiber, Fat, Fatty Acids, Cholesterol, Protein and Amino Acids*, underscores the value of nutrition even more.

Reading the headlines might lead you to believe that you need to worry only about cholesterol to steer clear of the heart-attack track or just increase your calcium intake for bone health. Actually, you need to think of the big picture because gearing your eating habits to avoid the disease of the year isn't enough. In this chapter I summarize and simplify information about nutrition and health—including emerging issues.

SIFTING THROUGH THE NUTRITION HEADLINES

If you ate according to the nutrition headlines, one week you would be strapping on an oat bran bag, and the next, dousing your toast with flaxseed oil.

It's as if your diet is the ball in the tennis match of nutrition research, with food companies cheering you on.

Despite the consensus from scientific bodies about dietary risk factors, a lot of confusion exists. One reason is that the exact mechanism of many diseases is still being researched. Also, scientists studying the same topic often use different methods and consequently get different results. For example, there still is not a universal method for determining dietary fiber in food.

Another problem is that association does not prove cause and effect. For example, hair dryer use, aluminum foil use, and the gross national product are all higher in populations with increased breast cancer rates! But there is no reason to believe that these factors cause cancer. The association is purely incidental.

Adding to the confusion is the "*New England Journal of Medicine* phenomenon." With all due respect to this prestigious medical journal, one study published in NEJM does not prove or disprove a theory. It's the preponderance of evidence, from many well-designed studies with similar conclusions, that counts. The real conflict is that science is evolutionary, focusing on process, whereas the media focuses on revolutionary results. And sometimes the results are not significant if you look at the method or process of the study design.

Even given the difficulties of scientific research, enough data have been confirmed to warrant changes for healthy living in the typical American or westernized diet. Keep in mind that further research may fine-tune these recommendations, as science is indeed evolutionary. Let's examine the recommendations more closely.

BUILDING A SOLID FOOD FOUNDATION

The following nutritional recommendations are based on information from several governmental and health organizations, including the U.S. Department of Agriculture, the National Academy of Sciences, the American Cancer Society, and the American Heart Association. For a concise summary of dietary recommendations from various organizations, see table 8.1.

More, More, More

Eating the right quantities of quality foods brings balance to your body. Too often consumers think more is better and end up eating too much of the wrong things. The following sections explain what you need more of and how to get it.

Fiber Most Americans fall very short in their fiber intake. The average American eats only about half of the necessary dietary fiber daily. Men need 30 to 38 grams of fiber each day, and women 21 to 25 grams. One very nice attribute of fiber is that you do not absorb its calories, but its presence in food helps contribute to feeling full. Fiber is a nondigestible component

TABLE 8.1 DISEASE PREVENTION CHART: KEY NUTRITIONAL RECOMMENDATIONS

Organization, policy document	Increase fruits and vegetables	Increase whole grains	Increase fiber	Moderate total fat	Lower saturated fat	Limit cholesterol
AICR/WCRF, Expert Panel Report, 1997	5 servings/ day	Yes	Yes	15-30% of total calories	—	—
American Cancer Society, 2002	> 5 servings/ day	Yes, prefer over refined grains	Yes	Yes	—	—
American Heart Association, 2000	> 5 servings/ day	Yes	Yes	< 30% of total calories	< 10% of calories. Limit trans fatty acids.	< 300 mg/day
DASH	> 8 servings/ day	Yes	Yes	Yes	Yes	Yes
DASH-Sodium	> 8 servings/ day	Yes	Yes	Yes	Yes	Yes
Dietary Guidelines for Americans, USDA and DHHS 2000	> 3 servings vegetables, > 2 servings fruit	Yes	Yes	Yes	Yes	Yes
Food Guide Pyramid, USDA	> 3 servings vegetables, > 2 servings fruit	Yes, several servings a day	Yes	30% of calories, 53-93 g/day	Yes	Yes
Healthy People 2010, DHHS 2000	> 3 servings vegetables, > 2 servings fruit	Yes, at least 3 whole grains	—	< 30% of calories	< 10% of calories	Implied
Institute of Medicine's Dietary Reference Intakes, 2002	—	—	Men: 30-38 g Women: 21-25 g	20-35% of total calories	Low as possible. Limit trans fatty acids.	Low as possible
National High Blood Pressure Education Program, 2002	Yes, eat a diet rich in fruits and vegetables	—	—	Yes	Yes	—

Organization, policy document	Limit sugar	Limit sodium	Moderate alcohol	Exercise	Maintain healthy weight
AICR/WCRF, Expert Panel Report, 1997	< 10% of total calories	< 6 g/day of salt	No alcohol recommended. If consumed at all, < 2 drinks for men and 1 for women.	If occupational activity is low or moderate, take an hour's brisk walk or similar exercise daily and also exercise for a total of at least one hour in a week.	Yes
American Cancer Society, 2002	Limit pastries, sweetened cereals, soft drinks, and sugars	—	Yes, 2 drinks for men, 1 drink per day for women	> 30 min on > 5 days/wk	Yes
American Heart Association, 2000	Yes	< 6 g/day of salt (< 2,400 mg/day of sodium)	Limit to 2 drinks for men and 1 for women	> 30 min/day	Yes
DASH	< 5 servings/wk	3,000 mg sodium	—	—	—
DASH-Sodium	< 5 servings/wk	1,500-2,400 mg sodium	—	—	—
Dietary Guidelines for Americans, USDA and DHHS 2000	Yes	Yes	Yes, 2 drinks for men, 1 drink per day for women	> 30 min/day	Yes
Food Guide Pyramid, USDA	< 6-18 tsp./day	Yes	Yes, 1-2 drinks/day	—	—
Healthy People 2010, DHHS 2000	--	< 2,400 mg sodium	Yes	> 30 min/day	Yes
Institute of Medicine's Dietary Reference Intakes, 2002	< 25% total calories from added sugar	—	—	1 hr/day	—
National High Blood Pressure Education Program, 2002	—	< 2.5 g sodium	Limit for men: < 2 drinks/day. Limit for women and lighter-weight persons: < 1 drinks/day	> 30 min/day of aerobic activity most days of the week	Yes

(continued)

TABLE 8.1 *(continued)*

Organization, policy document	Other recommendations
AICR/WCRF, Expert Panel Report, 1997	Choose predominantly plant-based diets rich in a variety of vegetables and fruits, pulses (legumes), and minimally processed starchy staple foods. Limit red meat to 3 oz. daily. Store, preserve, and prepare food safely. Do not eat charred food. Limit cured and smoked meats, and limit meat and fish grilled or broiled in a direct flame.
American Cancer Society, 2002	Limit red meats. Eat a variety of healthy foods, with an emphasis on plant sources.
American Heart Association	Eat at least 2 fish servings per week. Achieve and maintain a healthy eating pattern that includes foods from each of the major food groups. Replaced saturated fat with grains and unsaturated fat from vegetables, fish, legumes, and nuts. Include fat-free and low-fat milk products, fish, beans, skinless poultry, and lean meats. Choose fats and oils with < 2 g/tbsp. of saturated fat. Limit intake of foods high in calories or low in nutrition.
DASH, DASH-Sodium	Eat 5 servings per week of nuts, seeds, and dry beans. Eat at least 3 servings of low-fat or fat-free dairy foods.
Dietary Guidelines for Americans, USDA and DHHS 2000	Keep foods safe to eat. Use the Food Guide Pyramid.

Food Guide Pyramid, USDA	Specific servings for food groups:
	  Bread: 6-11
	  Vegetables: 3-5
	  Fruit: 2-4
	  Milk: 2-3
	  Meat: 5-7 oz.

Healthy People 2010, DHHS 2000	Increase calcium intake. Increase iron to reduce iron-deficiency anemia. Eat at least 1 serving of dark green or orange vegetables a day.

Institute of Medicine's Dietary Reference Intakes, 2002	Carbohydrates: 45-65% of calories, > 130 g/day
	Protein: 10-35% of calories
	Essential fatty acid minimums:
	  —Linoleic acid: 12 g/day for women, 17 g/day for men.
	  —Alpha-linolenic acid: 1.1 g/day for women, 1.6 g/day for men.

National High Blood Pressure Education Program, 2002	Eat low-fat dairy products. Maintain an adequate intake of dietary potassium (3,500 mg/day).

AICR = American Institute for Cancer Research

DASH = Dietary Approaches to Stop Hypertension I (original study)

DASH-Sodium = Dietary Approaches to Stop Hypertension II

WCRF = World Cancer Research Fund

found in plants, that is, fruits, vegetables, legumes, and whole grains. We lack the enzyme necessary to break down fiber in the body, so our bodies are unable to absorb fiber. And if you don't absorb a food, its calories can't contribute to your fat stores. Here's a fiber bonus: researchers estimate that if we doubled our current low fiber intake, we would absorb up to 130 fewer calories per day. Specifically, men who double their daily fiber intake from the U.S. average of 18 grams to 36 grams absorb 130 fewer calories per day. Women who double their fiber intake from 12 to 24 grams per day have 90 fewer calories to worry about.

Fiber has unique physiological properties that are health enhancing. The soluble portion of fiber helps lower blood cholesterol and stabilize blood sugar. Soluble fiber is found in oats, beans, fruits, and vegetables. Insoluble fibers, such as whole wheat, are associated with increased bulk and increased transit time through the digestive system.

A high-fiber diet also helps protect against diverticulosis, an abnormal out-pouching of the intestines. Imagine squeezing a long balloon like the ones clowns shape into animals. When pressure is applied, the balloon bulges out. Similarly, a low-fiber diet results in very low bulk stool that causes difficulties with elimination. Unfortunately, once these pouches are formed, food particles can get trapped there, resulting in painful inflammation called diverticulitis.

How do you increase fiber in your diet? Your first impulse may be to add bran or bran tablets, but the solution is not that simple. Different fibers act differently in the body. Therefore, to reap all the benefits of fiber, you need to eat a variety of types of fiber, preferably from food. Interestingly enough, the benefits of fiber may ultimately be from their source: food. High-fiber diets are typically high in fruits, vegetables, legumes, and whole grains—all which have not only fiber but other health-enhancing compounds such as phytochemicals. Here is how to increase your fiber:

- Eat five or more servings of both fruits and vegetables. Choose whole fruits and vegetables, rather than their juices, to push up fiber levels.

- Choose whole-grain products such as whole wheat bread, brown rice, or barley. Be sure to choose breads that list *whole* wheat flour as the first ingredient. Otherwise you may wind up with white-flour bread in disguise. Don't be fooled by the term *wheat flour,* which is merely white flour. (Since white flour comes from wheat via lots of processing, it's legal to list it as wheat flour on the ingredient label.) Aim for at least three whole grains a day.

- Beans are one of the naturally richest sources of fiber. Include them consistently three times a week (or more) to give your diet a great fiber boost. Compare the fiber content of a typical serving of bran versus cooked beans, shown in table 8.2.

- Don't rely on fiber supplements.

TABLE 8.2 FIBER CONTENT IN BRAN VERSUS BEANS

Food	Total fiber(g)	Soluble fiber (g)
1/3 cup oat bran, uncooked	4	2
1/3 cup rice bran	5.5	1
1/3 cup wheat bran	8	1
1 cup black beans	12	5
1 cup kidney beans	14	6
1 cup pinto beans	12	3

Adapted from *Plant Fiber in Foods* (2nd ed.) by J.W. Anderson, 1990, Lexington, KY: HCF Nutrition Research Foundation. Copyright 1990 by J.W. Anderson.

Fish   The protective power of fish is so beneficial that the American Heart Association recommends eating it at least twice a week. Fatty fish in particular, such as salmon and mackerel are rich in omega-3 fatty acids, of which most people don't get enough. Omega-3 fatty acids are a family of fats that are garnering a lot of research attention because they have so many varied and positive effects. Omega-3 fatty acids have been to shown to lower cancer risk, decrease fatal heart arrhythmias, decrease inflammation from arthritis, improve depression, and even reduce age-related dementia. But Americans typically don't get enough of these fats, which are found in fatty fish, flaxseed oil, soy foods, and walnuts.

Carbohydrates   With so many folks on high-protein fad diets, the belief that carbohydrates are inherently fattening is prevalent. Not so, not so! Of course, a large quantity of any food can contribute to making fat, but remember that carbohydrates are an essential nutrient, vital to well-being. We need at least 130 grams of carbohydrates a day. While this amount is quite easy get in your diet, it's not so easy if you are avoiding carbohydrates, which provide essential fuel to the body and the exclusive fuel of the brain. Aim

Give Soy a Try

The emerging connection between soy foods and disease prevention is quite broad—from lowering cholesterol to helping bone health and possibly preventing some types of cancer. Eating 25 grams of soy protein a day can help lower cholesterol. Don't worry if you are not a tofu kind of person. There are many convenient soy products in your regular grocery store: soy nuts, soy yogurt, soy cheese, edamame (fresh soybeans), and frozen foods such as soy pizza and meatless soy patties.

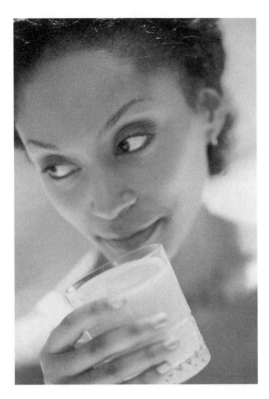

Orange juice is a great source of vitamin C and a tasty snack too!

for quality carbohydrates, found in whole grains, fruits, yogurt, starchy vegetables, milk, and beans.

Iron   Don't forget the iron! Vitamins and minerals are all important to health, but the number one nutrient deficiency worldwide and in the United States is iron-deficiency anemia. Classic symptoms include fatigue, but lack of iron can also hamper learning ability. Foods rich in iron include lean red meats, beans, dried fruits, and the dark meat of poultry.

Fruits and Vegetables   It is no secret that fruits and vegetables are truly a cornerstone of good health, with benefits that go beyond their rich nutrient and fiber content. Promising research shows that plant foods possess natural compounds that generate antioxidant action independently of their antioxidant nutrients, such as vitamin C. Researchers have developed a new tool that measures the antioxidant power, called the oxygen radical absorbance capacity (ORAC), of common vegetables and fruits. By measuring ORAC, researchers at Tufts University found that plant-based foods contain a natural antioxidant mixture that appears to be better than any single antioxidant nutrient (or even a mixture of nutrients). This "extra" antioxidant power combined with the nutrients already present in plants may explain why they are so healthful.

Before you get too confident that you are doing just fine in the fruits and vegetables department, the latest compelling research shows that optimal intake is at least eight servings (combined) a day! This finding comes from the DASH (Dietary Approaches to Stop Hypertension) trials. DASH is an eating pattern clinically proven to lower blood pressure, even in people without high blood pressure. DASH's impressive effect on blood pressure reduction was similar to that achieved in other studies through medication. This pattern of eating has also been shown to lower cholesterol and homocysteine. (Homocysteine is an amino acid that, when elevated in the blood, is related to increased risk of heart disease, stroke, and possibly Alzheimer's disease.) The DASH pattern of eating includes eating low-fat dairy foods and nuts, seeds, and legumes. The DASH studies gave a provocative reason to include these plant foods at least four to five times a week, but even more research has demonstrated that the health benefits of eating nuts include decreased risk of stroke and heart disease, lower cholesterol, and increased satiety. To see what a typical day of DASH eating looks like, see table 8.3.

Calcium   Calcium is the well-known champion of bone health, a nutrient that many people fail to get enough of. Solid research from the DASH studies shows that calcium-rich foods in the form of low-fat or nonfat dairy products also play an important role in lowering blood pressure. We need at least three calcium-rich foods a day. Yet reaching for a calcium supplement may not do the trick as far as blood pressure is concerned. Calcium supplements did not have the same effect on lowering blood pressure as the DASH diet. Two key tricks include eating nuts, seeds, and beans at least four to five times a week and increasing physical activity. The DASH studies gave a provocative reason to include these plant foods regularly, but even more research has demonstrated the health benefits of eating nuts including: decreased risk of stroke and heart disease, lower cholesterol, and increased satiety. Just about

TABLE 8.3 DASH EATING PATTERN

Food group	Servings	A serving is:
Grains	7 to 8 daily	1 slice bread; 1/2 cup cooked rice, pasta, or cereal
Vegetables	4 to 5 daily	1 cup raw leafy; 1/2 cup cooked; 6 oz. vegetable juice
Fruits	4 to 5 daily	1 medium; 1/4 cup dried; 1/2 cup fresh, frozen, or canned; 6 oz. juice.
Dairy, low-fat or fat-free	2 to 3 daily	1 cup milk or yogurt; 1 1/2 oz. cheese
Meats, poultry, and fish	2 or fewer daily	3 oz.
Nuts, seeds, and dry beans	4 to 5 per week	1/3 cup or 1 1/2 oz. nuts; 2 tbsp. or 1/2 oz. seeds; 1/2 cup cooked dry beans
Fats and oils	2 to 3 daily	1 tsp. tub margarine or vegetable oil; 1 tbsp. low-fat mayonnaise; 2 tbsp. light salad dressing
Sweets	5 per week	1 tbsp. sugar, jam, or maple syrup; 1/2 oz. jelly beans or hard candy; 8 oz. lemonade, fruit punch, sorbet, or ices

The DASH eating pattern is rich in fruits, vegetables, and low-fat dairy foods. It includes nuts, seeds, and dry beans at least five times a week but is low in saturated fat and total fat.

Adapted from NIH publication no. 98-4082, September 1998.

every dietary guideline recommends a minimum of at least 30 minutes of physical activity daily, and preferably 60 minutes a day. Keep in mind that this activity does not have to be done in one continuous session at a time. The most important tip is to find an active routine that you enjoy, whether it's walking or joining a gym.

Less, Less, Less

For a balanced diet it's important to eat less of the things that are not nutritionally beneficial. Following are suggestions for cutting back on the things that do more harm than good.

Fat   The most important fat guideline has to do with quantity and quality. Health authorities recommend that only 20 to 35 percent of our calories come from fat. These fats are best chosen from sources of high nutritional quality, which include polyunsaturated fats (such as corn or safflower oil), omega-3 fatty acids (flaxseed oil, walnuts, or salmon), and monounsaturated fats (such as canola oil or olive oil).

The type of fat you eat affects your blood cholesterol, and high cholesterol is a risk factor contributing to heart disease. Saturated fats have a profound effect in raising cholesterol levels. These fats are found in full-fat dairy products, all animal fats, and tropical oils (coconut oil, palm oil, and palm kernel oil). The body has no requirement for saturated fat, and it should constitute less than 10 percent of your daily calories (less is better). Table 8.4 shows how many grams of saturated fat you can eat without exceeding this 10 percent level.

The body also has no need for trans fatty acids, yet these fats are prevalent in fast foods and bakery products. This type of fat is created when hydrogen is added to an oil to make it harder (hydrogenated oil), as in stick-style margarine or vegetable shortening. Trans fatty acids may have a more deleterious

TABLE 8.4   MAXIMUM SATURATED FAT

Calories	Maximum saturated fat (g)*
1,200	13
1,500	16
1,800	20
2,100	23
2,400	26
2,700	30
3,000	33

*Artery-clogging saturated fat should not exceed 10 percent of your daily calories.

effect on blood cholesterol than even saturated fat, as they have a twofold negative consequence. Trans fatty acids raise LDL ("bad") cholesterol while they lower the protective HDL cholesterol.

Keep in mind, however, that our bodies need some fat. Not all fat is "bad." We require two essential fatty acids for health: linoleic acid and alpha-linolenic acid. In fact, alpha-linolenic acid in particular may confer additional health benefits, as it is an omega-3 fatty acid. Here are the minimum requirements for these essential fats:

Linoleic acid	Alpha-linolenic acid
Men: 14-17 g/day	Men: 1.6 g/day
Women: 11-12 g/day	Women: 1.1 g/day

Omega-3 fatty acids are a family of fats that are garnering a lot of research attention because they have so many varied and positive effects on our body. But Americans typically don't get enough of these fats which are found in fatty fish, flaxseed oil, soy foods, and walnuts.

Cholesterol   You get cholesterol two ways. Your liver makes cholesterol, and you get it from the foods that you eat. Only animal products contain cholesterol, such as egg yolks, butter, meats, poultry, fish, cheese, and other full-fat dairy products. One of the highest sources of cholesterol is egg yolks, which provide 215 milligrams of cholesterol (71 percent of the recommended maximum daily intake).

To keep your dietary cholesterol in check, make sure your daily intake of meat (anything with fins, fur, or feathers) does not exceed seven ounces, preferably down to four ounces. This is how you can limit your meat consumption easily:

- Replace meat-based meals with bean-based meals.
- Use meat as a condiment rather than as the "main event," as in dishes such as spaghetti or stir-fry.
- Limit meat to just one meal rather than two or three meals per day.
- Limit egg yolks, especially in cooking. Acquire the "poke-a-yoke" habit: treat eggs like olives and get rid of the yolk. Use two egg whites in place of each whole egg in cooking, or use egg substitute. By the way, most restaurants offer egg substitutes or egg whites on request.
- Lighten up the cheese. Make it a habit to use only lower-fat varieties (those with less than five grams of fat per ounce). This usually means holding the cheese when eating out.
- Use nonfat or low-fat dairy products.

Salt   High-sodium diets have been associated with high blood pressure and cancer of the stomach and esophagus. But until recently researchers had debated about recommending lower-sodium diets for healthy people.

The DASH-Sodium trials removed all doubts about the benefit of lowering sodium in everyone's diet. Your odds of getting high blood pressure during your lifetime are 90 percent! This statistic is based on research from the Framingham Heart Study. High blood pressure is one of seven proven major risk factors for heart disease that you can change.

The recommend maximum daily consumption of salt (sodium chloride) is six grams, which is equivalent to 2,400 milligrams of sodium daily. A healthier goal is 1,500 milligrams of sodium or less. "But I don't use salt," you may say. Most of the sodium in U.S. diets does not come from the salt shaker! About 75 percent of sodium is consumed in the form of processed foods. Only 15 percent of sodium intake is from salt added at the table or in cooking. Surprised? Consider that foods such as frozen waffles and instant pudding have about 500 milligrams of sodium per serving—and they don't even taste salty. Fast food is also notoriously high in sodium (see chapter 5). The following steps can help you reduce your sodium intake:

- Read food labels carefully and check for sodium content.
- Decrease your use of salty condiments such as soy sauce, steak sauce, pickles, and olives.
- Think spicy rather than salty. Reach for spices and herbs in cooking more often, and rely less on added salt. Try dry mustard, garlic powder, onion, lemon, cumin, dill, and other sodium-free seasonings.
- Limit consumption of cured and smoked meats; instead buy plain or oven-roasted meats.

Alcohol   Heavy drinkers are at risk for developing cancer of the mouth, larynx, esophagus, and liver. Alcohol also increases the risk for high blood pressure. For those who drink, the upper limit should be no more than two drinks a day for men and one drink a day for women. One drink is equivalent to

One 12-ounce can of beer

One glass of wine

1/2 ounce of hard liquor

If you are trying to reduce calories, alcohol is a good place to start. Of course, pregnant women should abstain from alcoholic beverages.

Sugar   Sugar and sweeteners supply very little in the way of nutrients (an exception is blackstrap molasses) but can add substantial calories. Hence they are commonly described as "empty calories." Americans eat an average 21 teaspoons of sugar per day. Even if you don't add sugar to your foods, consider that a typical 12-ounce soda has nine teaspoons of sugar and one granola bar has about four teaspoons of sugar. You can see how this adds up.

Fortunately, sugar is not linked with deadly diseases, although eating sweets is certainly related to dental caries. Try these tips to reduce your sugar intake:

- Choose canned fruits packed in their own juice or with no sugar added.
- Instead of soda, try mineral water, nonfat or low-fat milk, iced tea, or juice.
- Sweet tooth? Make each sweet count. Be sure to sit and savor, and try increasing the nutrient density by choosing foods with more nutritional value, such as hot chocolate made with nonfat milk, frozen yogurt, or a chocolate-covered strawberry.
- Reduce your added sugar by 25 percent; the food or beverage will still taste good but will have less sugar.
- Enhance the perception of sweetness by using sweet spices and extracts such as cinnamon, nutmeg, allspice, and vanilla.

CHAPTER 9

Supplementing a Healthy Diet

Feeling a little draggy? Need extra energy? Will popping some vitamins perk you up a little? Can supplements be an effective nutritional shortcut to optimal health? If you decide to take a supplement, which is best? When you are on the run, more often than not, normal fatigue (not due to illness) is related to the following:

- Inadequate sleep
- Not enough food (or the wrong types)
- Going long periods without eating
- Overtraining (exercise)
- Mental stress

Taking a vitamin supplement will not make up for sleep deprivation, stress, or lack of eating. If it were only that easy, I would be the first in line with my hand out and my mouth wide open. Although some vitamin and mineral deficiencies, such as iron deficiency anemia, can cause fatigue, vitamins themselves do not supply energy. Only carbohydrates, protein, and fat do. Vitamins help convert these energy-supplying nutrients into the biochemical form that the body needs.

If fatigue comes from burning the candle at both ends, your best solution is a combination of sleep, stress management (including setting limits for projects and your schedule), and mindful eating, rather than simply taking a supplement. Think of it this way: when endurance athletes want extra energy for performance, they are advised to load carbohydrates, not vitamins.

POPULAR MISCONCEPTIONS

An unhealthy diet with a vitamin and mineral supplement still remains an unhealthy diet. A supplement is no excuse for poor eating, but it can easily become a crutch if you are not careful. The core nutritional problem in this country is not one of deficits but rather excesses: too much saturated fat, too much cholesterol, and too much sodium. You have already seen that these particular dietary components have the most damaging effect on your health. A supplement will not counteract a diet that is high fat, high sodium, high cholesterol, or low fiber. Following are some popular misconceptions people have about vitamin and mineral supplements.

A good supplement will meet all your nutritional needs.

No such single supplement exists because everything you need could not fit into a gulp-size pill. In addition, many factors that enhance nutrient absorption are found only in foods.

Supplement companies can put only the known nutrients into their pills.

Some important nutrients and food factors, such as phytochemicals may not have been discovered or identified yet. For example, phytochemicals, compounds that occur naturally in plant foods, have been found to fight cancer, but scientists have barely scratched the surface of identifying them. Broccoli alone, for example, has about 34 phytochemicals. But until they are identified and isolated, phytochemicals cannot be added to supplements. And even if added to a supplement, they might not be effective. For example, a study conducted in the Carotenoid and Health Lab at Tufts University demonstrated that a pill containing six grams of lutein did not have the same effect as a diet containing the same amount of lutein. The lutein-rich spinach diet phase of the study increased blood levels of lutein by more than 40 percent compared to the same amount of lutein in pill form. The researchers concluded that the dietary lutein was much more available to the body than the pill form. It was also significantly less costly to get lutein from the diet.

Supplements labeled "natural" are better than other supplements.

The most natural form in which a vitamin can be found is food! To get a vitamin or mineral into pill form requires many extraction processes and then condensation into a tablet or capsule; this is far from natural. The term *natural* is not well defined and is often just a marketing gimmick to imply unsubstantiated benefits or safety.

Nutritional supplements are safe.

As toxicologists are fond of saying, it's the dose that makes the poison or cure. Nutrients in high levels can be dangerous. For example, the mineral iron can be fatal in large doses. That's why you the see the warning labels on children's vitamins. Iron overdose is one of the most common causes of poisoning in children.

MEGADOSING

Some people unknowingly play Russian roulette with their metabolism. Despite the fact that vitamins and minerals sound so natural and healthy, they are not necessarily innocuous. Megadosing can be hazardous to your health, which is a sad irony because many people think they are improving their health by taking high doses of supplements. More, in the case of vitamins and minerals, is not better.

The body handles high doses of nutrients similarly to drugs. As a result, extra metabolic stress is placed on the liver and kidneys. It may take years for the damage to show up. I'm amazed at how often my new clients have no idea of the dosages of the vitamins and minerals they take. Most nutrients have a Tolerable Upper Intake Level (UL) set by the Food and Nutrition Board of the Institute of Medicine. The UL was established to help people avoid adverse effects and imbalances from excessive nutrient intakes. To see how your current supplement stacks up, see table 9.1.

TABLE 9.1 TOLERABLE UPPER INTAKE LEVEL (UL) FOR MINERALS AND VITAMINS

Minerals	UL Men and women* ≥ 19 yr.	DRI Men ≥ 19 yr.	DRI Women* ≥ 19 yr.
Boron, mg/day	20	—	—
Calcium, mg/day	2,500	1,000-1,200	1,000-1,200
Chromium, μg/day	**	30-35	20-25
Copper, μg/day	1,000	900	900
Fluoride, mg/day	10	4	3
Iodine, mg/day	1,100	150	150
Iron, mg/day	45	8	18*** 8****
Magnesium, mg/day	350	420	310-320
Manganese, mg/day	11	2.3	1.8
Molybdenum, μg/day	2,000	45	45
Nickel, μg/day	1,000	—	—
Phosphorus, mg/day	3,000-4,000	700	700
Selenium, μg/day	400	55	55
Vanadium, mg/day	1.8	—	—
Zinc, mg/day	40	11	8
Vitamins			
Biotin, μg/day	**	30	30
Choline, mg/day	3,500	550	425
Folate, μg/day	1,000	400	400
Niacin, mg/day	35	16	14

(continued)

TABLE 9.1 *(continued)*

Pantothenic acid, mg/day	**	5	5
Vitamin A, μg/day	3,000	900	700
Vitamin B$_1$ (thiamin), μg/day	**	1.2	1.1
Vitamin B$_{12}$ (cobalamin), μg/day	**	2.4	2.4
Vitamin B$_2$ (riboflavin), mg/day	**	1.3	1.1
Vitamin B$_6$ (pyridoxine), mg/day	100	1.3-1.7	1.3-1.5
Vitamin C (ascorbic acid), mg/day	2,000	90	75
Vitamin D, μg/day	50	5-15	5-15
Vitamin E, mg/day	1,000	15	15
Vitamin K, μg/day	**	120	90

The Dietary Reference Intake (DRI) in the last columns is given for comparison. The DRI is a new reference value that has replaced the Recommended Dietary Allowance (RDA).

* Not including pregnant or lactating women.

** Due to lack of data, the UL could not be established.

*** Ages 19-50

**** Ages ≥ 51

Adapted from the Dietary Reference Intakes (Food and Nutrition Board, 2001).

TOXICITY

It is widely known that fat-soluble vitamins, especially vitamins A and D, can be toxic in large amounts because they are stored in the body. Levels of three to five times the Recommended Dietary Intake (RDI) may cause birth defects when taken by a mother during pregnancy.

Some water-soluble vitamins have also been shown to be hazardous in large amounts. For example, vitamin B6 has been shown to cause symptoms of paralysis and other dysfunctions of the nervous system in women taking large doses. One of the best examples of toxicity in high doses is the water-soluble vitamin niacin, which also has been legitimately classified as a drug. Niacin is considered a therapeutic drug when given in large doses to help lower triglycerides and cholesterol. But as drug, niacin also has side effects, such as gout, liver problems, aggravation of peptic ulcers, and elevated blood sugar, that have been documented in clinical trials. Therefore, niacin to help control triglycerides or cholesterol should be taken under the supervision of a physician who can watch for any side effects.

Robbing Peter to Pay Paul

One way supplements can hurt your nutritional status is by robbing Peter to pay Paul, that is, high doses of one nutrient displacing another. For example, large doses of zinc inhibit copper absorption. High-calcium supplements can impair iron absorption. Large doses of the essential amino acid leucine can inhibit the uptake of another essential amino acid, isoleucine. This why supplements that provide a single vitamin or mineral, such as just zinc or just vitamin B_6, can especially upset your metabolic machinery. They represent a hit-or-miss approach to nutrition that throws you off balance.

Nutrients must be kept in balance, or you may induce a deficiency. That's unlikely to happen if you are getting your nutrients through nature's best package, food. If supplementation is necessary, I discuss how to go about it sensibly later in this chapter.

In the infamous Beta-Carotene and Retinol Efficacy Trial (CARET) involving 18,000 former smokers and workers exposed to asbestos, researchers had to halt the study midway (after four years) because the combination of beta-carotene and vitamin A supplements actually increased the risk of lung cancer in smokers by 28 percent! The researchers concluded, "The results of the trial are troubling." Until then, it had been widely accepted that a diet rich in beta-carotene or vitamin A had preventive health advantages. The key word here is food. In supplement form, these substances were hazardous to smokers.

Minerals can also be quite toxic. A recent zinc toxicity case was reported in the *Journal of Pediatric Hematology/Oncology.* A teenage boy was taking zinc supplements for his acne but was seeing no results, so he upped his intake to 300 milligrams per day. (The recommended level for teens 14 to 18 years old is 11 milligrams, and the Tolerated Upper Intake Level is 34 milligrams.) He ended up with anemia, extreme fatigue, and neutropenia (a condition in which a type of white blood cell, neutrophils, is abnormally low). He stopped taking the zinc. After two weeks, his zinc blood levels were still two to three times greater than normal. At four months he was almost fully recovered, although at six months his zinc levels were still slightly elevated above normal.

These are some other adverse effects to consider:

➧ Supplements may interact with prescription medication and over-the-counter medicines. For example, vitamins E and K can interfere with the blood thinner Coumadin. A heart medication study of 160 patients with heart disease showed that antioxidants caused an adverse interaction with the cholesterol-lowering medication Zocor plus niacin. Antioxidants in this situation lowered HDL ("good") cholesterol and interfered with the HDL-raising effects of the medication.

*Some supplements can have an undesirable effect during surgery. Therefore, it is important to fully inform your doctor about which supplements you are taking, including the dose.

*The supplement industry is self-monitored and is not required to report adverse effects from supplements. Therefore, adverse effects of supplements are underreported.

SUPPLEMENTAL NEEDS

Who can benefit from taking a supplement? It depends on who you ask! Two recent scientific literature reviews in the *Journal of the American Medical Association* make a strong case for all adults to use a daily multivitamin supplement. The national advocacy group Center for Science in the Public Interest (CSPI) recommends that everyone take a Centrum-like multivitamin and mineral supplement. Meanwhile, the American Dietetic Association recommends that decisions about supplements should be tailored to an individual's needs.

There is general agreement that certain groups are most likely to benefit from supplements (as established by the Food and Nutrition Board of the Institute of Medicine):

*All women capable of becoming pregnant should get 400 micrograms of folic acid from supplements or fortified foods to prevent birth defects, specifically neural tube defects.

*People older than 50 years, who are at risk of malabsorbing vitamin B_{12}, can benefit by getting this vitamin from supplements or fortified foods.

*Calcium and vitamin D supplements are recommended for those who avoid or minimize dairy products.

Additionally, I believe the following groups can also benefit from a supplement (but not a megadose):

*Devout vegetable haters

*Perpetual dieters

*Strict vegetarians or those who do not eat an entire food group

*Elderly people who have difficulty eating and preparing food

*Frequent meal skippers

Even the American Dietetic Association concedes that there is little evidence of harm from a multivitamin and mineral supplement in amounts that do not exceed 100 percent of the Dietary Reference Intake (DRI). Given the American Medical Association's and CSPI's recommendations, I see no problem in routinely taking a general multivitamin and mineral supplement.

Keep in mind that minerals are no less important than vitamins; they are both essential classes of nutrients, so you might as well go for a broad-spectrum multivitamin and mineral supplement, such as Centrum or an equivalent.

CHOOSING A SUPPLEMENT SENSIBLY

Here some guidelines to help you choose a supplement. Keep in mind that supplements can't replace the hundreds of food factors and phytochemicals found in whole foods, nor do they make up for poor eating habits.

1. Choose a multivitamin and mineral supplement rather than the bullet approach of single-nutrient pills. However, most of these once-daily supplements have very little calcium, so you may need to take a separate calcium supplement if you are falling short in low-fat dairy foods or calcium-fortified foods (such as orange juice).

2. Avoid megadose supplements. Most of the toxicity cases are from high-dose supplements. Check the Daily Value of the nutrients listed on the label of the supplement. Be sure that it provides about 100 percent of the Daily Value of all the nutrients it supplies. Also keep in mind any fortified foods that you may be eating on a regular basis, such as cereal, and be sure that the combination of these fortified foods and your supplement don't exceed the Tolerable Upper Intake Level (UL; refer to table 9.1 for these numbers).

3. Check the expiration date. Vitamins especially can lose their potency over time. If the supplement doesn't have an expiration date, don't buy it.

4. Look for the USP stamp of approval on the label. The U.S. Pharmacopeia (USP) is a testing organization that makes sure supplements meet the minimal standard for strength, purity, and dissolution (ability to be dissolve and be absorbed).

5. If you have allergies or food intolerances, check the inert ingredients. For example, lactose, a common inert ingredient, is a problem if you are lactose intolerant. Starch is a common ingredient that may contain wheat and is a problem if you have a wheat allergy or celiac disease.

6. If you take a calcium supplement, don't take it at the same time as an iron-containing supplement. Calcium interferes with iron absorption.

7. It's a good idea to check with your physician before taking a supplement.

DECIPHERING THE SUPPLEMENT LABEL

Sometimes labels are more frustrating than helpful. With the following breakdown of the elements on a supplement label (and some that aren't), the next time you glance at the back of the bottle, you'll know what you're getting.

◢ **Percentage Daily Value (%DV)**—This is one of the most useful bits of information on a supplement label; it tells you what percentage of the Daily

Value for nutrients the supplement supplies. For example, 50% DV for iron tells you that you are getting half of your daily iron needs in one dose of the supplement. This allows you to size up a supplement without having to memorize the Dietary Reference Intake (DRI)—just check the percentages. In general, you should not exceed 100 percent of the Daily Value without supervision from your physician or a registered dietitian. If you are malnourished or have a medical condition, you may need higher levels than the DRI.

➤ **Dietary Reference Intake (DRI)**—You won't see DRI on the supplement label, but it's helpful to understand this relatively new term in the field of nutrition. The DRI reflects the Institute of Medicine's Food and Nutrition Board's determination of an adequate amount of a nutrient at various life stages for each sex. It replaces the RDA (Recommended Dietary Allowance). The DRI is used mostly in nutrition assessment and planning.

➤ **Tolerable Upper Intake Level (UL)**—This is the highest daily intake of a nutrient that does not cause adverse reactions. For some nutrients, there was not enough data to establish a UL, but this does not mean that a high dose poses no risk of adverse effects. You won't see UL on the supplement label, but it's helpful to be aware of the UL so that you can make sure that your supplement in addition to the fortified foods you eat doesn't exceed the maximum recommended levels for nutrients.

FURTHER READING AND USEFUL WEB SITES

To keep up to date on supplements and nutrient requirements, check out these resources:

1. National Institutes of Health, Office of Dietary Supplements (www.odp.od.nih.gov/ods)

    This is a superb Web site full of recent relevant studies on various supplements. Especially helpful is the International Bibliographic Information on Dietary Supplements (IBIDS), which summarizes key studies.

2. Dietary Reference Intake Reports (www.nap.edu)

    Free access to the Dietary Reference Intake reports, although the size of each report can be cumbersome.

3. MedWatch (www.fda.gov/medwatch/how.htm)

    You can report any suspected adverse effects from the use of dietary supplements to the Food and Drug Administration at this Web site. You can also call 800-332-1088, toll-free.

While this book is targeted toward health professionals, it is also helpful for consumers. (It was recommended as a top pick by the *Wall Street Journal*.) It lists alphabetically many supplements and their current known efficacy. It provides solid research summaries and was reviewed by a panel of experts from the American Dietetic Association for accuracy before publication.

CHAPTER **10**

Healthy Choices for Busy Families

*Only 1 percent of children 2 to 19 years old meet all of the
Food Guide Pyramid guidelines.*
—Journal of the American Dietetic Association

If Mom and Dad are on the run, who's feeding the kids? Let's not forget that children have busy schedules, too—be it dance lessons, soccer practice, or weekend baseball tournaments—which means that the whole family is often on the run. The kids may be coming home to an empty house and preparing their own snacks or meals. Even when parents are home, children can be subject to the same eating challenges as adults face, from frozen meals to fast foods. In addition, kids face hurdles created by a food industry aimed just at children, which also makes it hard on parents!

GIMMICKS FOR KIDS

Unlike adults, kids are wooed by the food industry with toys and trinkets. Happy Meal sales accounted for 20 percent of U.S. purchases at McDonald's, adding up to a whopping $3.5 billion in annual revenue.

For years the kid food wars were primarily the domain of the cereal aisles. But the specialty kid market has grown—from edible cartoon characters to baseball cards buried in the food. Look at what the specialty kid food industry has to offer:

- Flintstones vitamins
- Dino Buddies frozen chicken nuggets
- Scooby-Doo cereal
- McDonald's Happy Meals
- Hot Wheels fruit snacks

Get the picture? The trend is for best-selling toys, cartoons, or movies to become food, of sorts. Too often this leads to a lot of razzle without the important nutritional dazzle. That's unfortunate because the growing years are a critical time for developing healthful eating habits. And statistics show some rather shocking facts about our children's health. For instance, in the United States, childhood obesity doubled over the past decade, and 15 percent of six- to nine-year-olds are overweight. More kids than ever are developing type 2 diabetes, a condition that usually occurs in adulthood.

In this chapter we will delve into how parents can help their children eat healthier, even when eating fast food, frozen food, or other convenience foods. We'll also look at snacking and children's vitamins. First, we'll go over guidelines to help your child develop healthy eating habits regardless of where he or she eats.

PARENT PARADOX

All too often I have counseled well-meaning parents who want their kids to eat healthfully but who do this by imposing rigid eating rules that end up having undesirable effects. Strict eating rules can backfire by causing kids to

- be out of touch with their own inner cues of hunger,
- eat snacks when they are not hungry,
- overeat when mom or dad is not looking,
- sneak food,
- eat *more* of the very food that is restricted, or
- become overweight.

A 1996 study from child feeding expert Leann L. Birch underscores this problem. The study demonstrated that a parent's use of restrictive feeding practices not only promotes eating in the absence of hunger, it actually triggers the consumption of the particular restricted food! Many other compelling studies have demonstrated this paradox.

It's important to allow your child to listen to internal hunger and fullness cues. This also means not telling your child to clean his or her plate. Children need to learn to become the experts on their own bodies' biological cues. Otherwise, your child's development of self-regulating eating cues is undermined, which in turn makes him or her more vulnerable to eating when not hungry *and* eating larger amounts of food. Instead, your child's desire to eat easily becomes triggered by the food environment. This includes the mere presence of food, size of the portion, and social context, not to mention the ever-present food marketing tactics that make food captivating.

One study demonstrated how one environmental factor, portion size, can influence kids. When four- to six-year-olds were served a double portion of food, their intake increased by 60 percent. Yet, two- to three-year-old children who were served small or large portions of food ate the same amount, regardless of portion size. Children at this age have not yet been as tainted by environmental triggers to eat, including parents' food rules. Given ever-growing food portions, it's even more important to encourage your child's sense of internal eating cues.

What about the picky eater? Don't be overly concerned about food jags; they are normal in children. Keep in mind that younger kids are especially reluctant to try new foods; this behavior, called neophobia, is natural. It takes an average 8 or 10 times of *tasting* (not just seeing) a food before a child will accept it. Children are capable of learning to accept and like a wide variety of foods. It just takes gentle, repeated exposure to a variety of foods.

What's a Parent to Do?

Here are some guidelines to help your child develop healthy eating habits:

- Encourage your child to focus on his or her own hunger and fullness as a guide to when eating should start and end.
- Create a positive environment for eating.
- Offer portion sizes appropriate to your child's needs.
- Offer a variety of foods.
- Have regular meals and snacks.
- Take time to relax and savor the eating experience when possible.
- Set a good example. Your actions are far more powerful than your words.
- Offer new food tasting experiences.
- Don't use food as a reward or bribe.
- Eat family meals together when possible.
- Consider the timing of meals. While an adult can easily delay eating, kids have difficulty if a meal is delayed too long and end up irritable and overhungry.

SNACKING

Snacking is vital for growing children to ensure that they get enough calories to support their growth. It's hard for kids to meet all of their nutritional needs in three meals because of their small stomachs and appetites. Choosing healthy snacks is the key, yet how does an ordinary snack pack of carrot sticks compete with a "superpower" cartoon character on a box of cookies or cereal? Keep the pointers in mind in table 10.1.

TABLE 10.1 SNACKING IDEAS

Instead of	Try
Candy	Peanut butter on apple wedges, bananas, or celery; peanut butter and jelly sandwich; dried fruit; trail mix
Chips, crackers	Light corn tortilla chips, light popcorn, whole-grain crackers, whole wheat bread sticks, nuts
Cookies	Graham crackers, oatmeal cookies, whole wheat apricot bars, whole wheat fig bars, vanilla wafers, gingersnaps
Cream-filled snack cakes	Sweet breads, such as banana nut, pumpkin, zucchini, poppy seed, apricot, or raisin
Dip	Plain yogurt with your favorite dip mix, such as ranch-style, added
Doughnuts	Variety bagels, such as raisin, apple, cinnamon, blueberry, or strawberry
Gelatin	Prepare with 100 percent fruit juice instead of water and any canned fruit
Ice cream sundae	Frozen yogurt or low-fat ice cream topped with berries; frozen juice bars
Pie	Baked fruit (e.g., an apple or a pear sprinkled with a little cinnamon and brown sugar); pudding made with nonfat or low-fat milk and topped with crushed graham crackers
Soda	Fruit fizzies: 3 parts juice to 1 part mineral water. Grape, orange, and cherry juices work well. Be sure to use 100 percent fruit juice.

TAKING TIME FOR TEENS

Teens are especially on the run. They often juggle school, practices, games, clubs, homework, part-time jobs, and friendships. When they arrive home, usually before their parents, they often head straight to the fridge. Teens like anything fast that they can eat with their fingers on the way out the door to their next event. I work with a lot of teens in my counseling practice, and the last thing they want is to be told what to do by their parents. Parental preaching (however well-intended) does not work with this age group. Here are a couple of key strategies:

- Don't try to control what your teen is allowed to eat, but offer healthy options for snacks and mealtimes.
- Stock the pantry with healthy snacks, including dried fruit, nuts, low-fat chips, whole wheat bread.

- Stock the fridge with nonfat yogurt, lean deli meats, low-fat cheese, ready-to-eat baby carrots, corn tortillas.
- Keep a fruit bowl within easy reach: it's eye-catching, quick, and easy.
- Try to coordinate schedules to eat family dinner together. Research shows that teens who eat dinner with their families have healthier diets.

Teens on the Run and Eating Disorders

Sometimes being "too busy" to eat or skipping meals masks an eating disorder. Eating disorders affect both girls and boys and can have life-threatening consequences. Here are some warning signs and symptoms:

- Is never seen eating
- Expresses worry about getting fat
- Exercises excessively
- Is preoccupied with weight and food
- Makes excuses for not eating
- Avoids many foods or expresses fear about eating certain foods
- Has a change (loss or gain) in weight
- Seems tired and withdrawn
- Weighs self often
- Disappears into the bathroom after eating
- Is irritable and has mood swings
- Showers after meals
- Is constantly dieting or restricting foods under the guise of "healthy eating"
- Drinks a lot of caffeinated beverages (diet cola, coffee, and coffee drinks)

   For more information, see the National Eating Disorders Association Web site, www.nationaleatingdisorders.org.

BUYING KID-FRIENDLY FOODS

It's easy to fall into the same trap when shopping for kids as it is for adults: fast, convenient, prepackaged, and ready-to-go. However, when eating at a restaurant or cruising the grocery aisles, remember to use the same caution with what you buy for your children as you do for yourself. The habits that you instill in them in youth will have an outstanding effect when they're on their own.

Grocery Stores and Delis

Navigating the aisle of the grocery store for kid's meals—whether frozen, canned, or the deli lunch packs—can be just as challenging as ordering fast-food meals. While most of these options are quite convenient, they unfortunately don't contribute much in the way of nutrition. One of the biggest culprits is in the deli section, so let's start there.

Deli Lunch Packs   One of the poorest meal finds for kids is the "lunch packs" found in the deli section. Most are very high in sodium, fat, and calories but low in fiber (see table 10.2). A newcomer is Lunchables Fun Fuel by Oscar Mayer. Although they still are high in sodium and low in fiber, they are much improved over the traditional Lunchables. Each Fun Fuel has 100 percent fruit juice and reduced-fat versions of cheese, yogurt, and mayonnaise, and the meats are lean: white chicken, turkey breast, and lean ham.

For convenience, buy the school lunch; at least it has to conform to national health standards set by USDA, and it's quicker than a trip to the grocery store. Consider packing lunches. Too pressed for time to pack lunch? Try packing it the night before and keeping it in the refrigerator. Better yet, get your child involved and let him or her pack part or all of the lunch. If you still want to get a deli lunch pack for your child, Fun Fuel is the better choice.

Canned and Frozen Cuisine   One of the challenges of frozen kid's meals is that they usually come with dessert. The meals can be also be high in sodium. The best strategy is to buy a "healthy" adult meal, such as Healthy Choice, and a separate convenient dessert of your own choosing, such as frozen yogurt, frozen juice bars, or low-fat pudding. Canned cuisine for kids is not a complete meal, just an entree. If you buy these canned foods, be sure to round out the meal by adding milk, easy vegetables such as baby carrots (no preparation necessary), and some fresh fruit (make it easy: get the fresh diced melon bowl in the produce section). Be sure to choose lower-sodium entrees (see tables 10.3 and 10.4).

Fast Food and Restaurants

Keeping up with the latest, greatest Happy Meal toy is a test not only of your patience but also of your wallet. Everyone markets to children—from the movie and television industries to restaurants and fast-food joints. What starts as a plain hamburger, fries, and a small soda turns into free advertisement for the latest Disney hit when you throw in a plastic figurine. While your kids get wrapped up in the toy, you need to watch what they eat!

TABLE 10.2 KID'S DELI MEALS

Item	Serving size	Calories	Protein (g)	Carbohy-drate (g)	Fiber (g)	Fat (g)	Saturated fat (g)	Sodium (mg)
Lunchables								
Pizza	1 package	470	16	65	2	17	8	750
Ultimate Nachos	1 package	800	9	107	6	38	9	1,620
Low-Fat Cracker Stackers	1 package	360-390	16	54-56	< 1	10-11	5	1,260-1,310
Burgers	1 package	460	14	67	1	15	9	1,030
Lunchables Fun Fuel								
Chicken Wraps	1 package	440	17	64	3	13	5	860
Ham Wraps	1 package	430	16	64	2	13	5	1,050
Turkey Bagels	1 package	420	16	64	2	10	4	830
Ham Bagels	1 package	410	16	64	2	40	4.5	890
Lunch Makers								
Loco Nachos	3.4 oz. food + 8 fl. oz. drink	370	4	59	4	13	2.5	730
Pizza	3.5 oz. food + 8 fl. oz. Drink	440	10	69	4	13	5	660
Cracker Crunchers	2.6 oz. food + 8 fl. oz. drink	360	10	48	1	14	7-8	850-860

TABLE 10.3 KID'S CANNED CUISINE

Item	Serving size	Calories	Protein (g)	Carbohy-drate (g)	Fiber (g)	Fat (g)	Saturated fat (g)	Sodium (mg)
Hormel Kid's Kitchen	1 container	140-320	8-12	18-37	1-7	4-16	1.5-8	720-1,000
Spaghettios	1 cup	180-240	6-11	30-36	3-5	1-10	0.5-3.5	600-990
Chef Boyardee	1 cup	200-300	5-11	32-43	0-4	0.5-13	0-5	780-1,290

TABLE 10.4 KID'S FROZEN CUISINE

Item	Serving size	Calories	Protein (g)	Carbohy-drate (g)	Fiber (g)	Fat (g)	Saturated fat (g)	Sodium (mg)
Kid's Cuisine (ConAgra Foods)	7.35-10.6 oz. (1 meal)	400-560	10-17	50-71	5-7	16-24	4-10	610-1,000
Stouffer's Maxaroni	19 oz. (1 serving)	390	16	44	2	17	7	1,160

Fast-Food Kid's Meal Packs Probably no other food industry packs as much fun and hype into eating as the fast-food industry. A fast-food kid's meal is a barrage of toys, fun packaging, games on the box, and movie promotions—plus playgrounds at many of the chains. Some have even put in free video game stations to keep the kids coming. Ever wonder why? The tiniest consumer has a lot of buying power because parents usually eat where their children eat.

Let's take a look at what the fast-food chains are packaging for kids. Generally, there is a choice of entree, such as a hamburger, cheeseburger, or chicken nuggets. Here's a typical example, a McDonald's Happy Meal including entree, small fries, and child-size orange drink:

Meal	Calories	Fat (g)	Saturated fat (g)	Sodium (mg)
Happy Meal with hamburger	610	20	6	725
Happy Meal with four chicken nuggets	540	23	5	595
Happy Meal with cheeseburger	660	24	8	965
Mighty Kids Meal with double hamburger	710	28	9	755
Mighty Kids Meal with double cheeseburger	810	37	14	1385
Mighty Kids Meal with six chicken nuggets	640	30	6	815

One problem with these packaged meals is that most automatically include fries and a soft drink. This can easily condition a child to want fries every time he or she orders in a fast-food place, even without the special kid package. If the kids are fond of fries, there's no harm in eating them occasionally, but it's best that fries do not become a routine order.

Fortunately, there have been some positive changes in some kid's meals. Kudos to KFC for including applesauce as part of the kid's meal and for offering a variety of sides from which to choose. McDonald's has other menu add-ons for kids, including Danimals Drinkable Lowfat Yogurt and reduced-fat ice cream.

As a parent or caregiver, you can get into a tug of war with a child who is pleading for a Happy Meal. Here are some strategies to win the battle, which I have used with my own children:

- If you buy a kid's meal, request milk or juice for the beverage rather than the typical soda. Most restaurants will accommodate you, although you may have to pay the difference in the price for the beverage.

- Of the typical entree choices (hamburger, cheeseburger, or chicken nuggets), the small hamburger is the best choice, believe it or not. It is the lowest in fat.

- Don't automatically order the kid's meal when driving through the fast-food outlet. Rather, order something different each time, or your child will learn to expect the kid's meal.

- If your child is more interested in visiting a particular fast-food place because of the hot toy that is being promoted, the healthiest option is to buy the toy separately, sans meal. Many restaurants provide that option.

- If your wants to order from the "big kid's" menu, it's best to stay with the smaller kid's meal and add some healthier sides, such as a baked potato, applesauce, yogurt, salad, or corn on the cob when available. See figure 10.1 for the best kid's meals at various fast-food chains.

Restaurant Kid's Meals   As challenging as restaurant eating can be for adults, it can more difficult for kids. Quite often the children's menu is limited and offers nowhere near the variety of foods of the adult menu. Most of these meals don't include vegetables or fruit, but there's never a shortage of french fries. In fact, it is common for national restaurant chains' kid's lunch and dinner menus to include french fries with four out of five kid's entrees. Here's what I found when I surveyed the kid's lunch/dinner menus of a few national restaurant chains:

- Carrows included french fries for 4 out 6 kids' entrees
- Chili's included french fries for 4 out 6 kids' entrees
- Denny's included french fries for 4 out 5 kids' entrees
- Red Robin included french fries for 4 out 7 kids' entrees

A good restaurant strategy is to make special requests. Keep in mind that the restaurant industry is service based and usually very accommodating.

FAST-FOOD KIDDIE PACKS

Listed below are the kid meal options. The entree with the asterisk is the better choice. In most instances, you can purchase the toy separately. Also, try substituting milk or orange juice (usually at no extra charge).

Arby's Adventure Meal

One Junior Roast Beef sandwich*

One small order of Homestyle Fries, Potato Cakes, or Curly Fries

Burger King Kids Meal

Hamburger,* cheeseburger, or four Chicken Tenders

French fries

Carl's Jr. Cool Kids Combo

Hamburger,* cheeseburger, four Chicken Stars, or two Chicken Breast Tender Strips

French fries

KFC Laptop Meals

Two Colonel's Crispy Strips, drumstick,* or Popcorn Chicken (where available)

One side dish (macaroni and cheese, mashed potatoes and gravy,* corn on the cob,* potato wedges, barbecue baked beans,* green beans,* potato salad, or coleslaw)

Applesauce

Fruit by the Foot

McDonald's Happy Meal

Hamburger,* cheeseburger, or four McNuggets

French fries

McDonald's Mighty Kids Meal

Double hamburger*, double cheeseburger, or six McNuggets

French fries

Taco Bell

Bean burrito* or two hard beef tacos

Nacho chips and cheese

Wendy's

Hamburger,* cheeseburger, or four Crispy Chicken Nuggets

French fries

Soft drink or Frosty (you can substitute milk at some locations)

Toy (not available for separate purchase)

Figure 10.1 Healthy fast-food choices are available for kids if you know where to look.

If they hear a request often enough, they might add it to the menu. Here are some healthy special requests:

- Vegetables or fruit instead of french fries
- Milk or orange juice instead of soda
- Grilled chicken rather than nuggets
- Grilled shrimp skewers or grilled fish rather than fish sticks

You can also simply split your entree with your child and order side dishes to complete your child's meal. Some good side dishes are baked beans, vegetables, fruit salad, corn on the cob, baked potato, mashed potatoes, watermelon wedge, and rice.

CHILDREN'S VITAMINS

Flintstones, Scooby-Doo, Pokemon—sounds like a Saturday morning television lineup. But these are typical brand names in the competitive chewable vitamin market for kids. Many of these cartoon supplements contain only vitamins, not minerals. But minerals are no less important than vitamins; they are essential nutrients too.

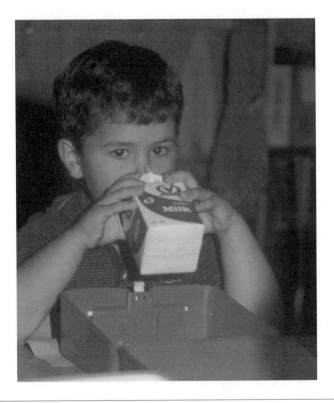

Forget the soda—get milk! It's better for the bones.

While it is possible to get the essential nutrients through food, the reality is that only 1 percent of children 2 to 19 years old meet all the Food Guide Pyramid guidelines. A multivitamin and mineral supplement can be a nice adjunct while children build a healthy eating base. However, you need to be cautious because so many children's foods, such as cereals, juices, and energy bars, are fortified with vitamins and minerals. And too much of a vitamin or mineral can be *toxic*. Here are some guidelines for supplement use:

- Remember, supplements are not a shortcut to, nor do they teach the foundation of, good lifelong eating habits.
- Choose a supplement that does not exceed 100 percent of the Daily Value that is listed under the Supplement Facts on the bottle.
- Stick with a multivitamin and mineral pill rather than a potpourri of single-nutrient pills.
- Be sure to check the dosage directions. For children two and three years old, this usually means taking only half a tablet.
- Store vitamins out of reach: they can be toxic, but they taste good.

SAVORING TIME TOGETHER

In the past, the evening meal was an opportunity for families to enjoy time together. In our busy lives today, we need to remember that making time for the family is important. Mealtime is a wonderful opportunity for family communication. Some families have found that the best time to eat together is in the morning. Find what works for you. Consider making a lunch or dinner date with your child; then enjoy a special meal together with no distractions.

We need to be careful not to impose our hurried eating on our children. Allow plenty of time for kids to eat (regardless of age), even if it means getting up an extra 15 minutes earlier because your child likes to savor his or her cereal. Although I see no problem with an adult's eating while walking in a tight schedule, this can be dangerous for a child because of the risk of choking.

Fueling for Sports and Fitness

*"I teach four to five aerobics classes a day and don't have
time to eat lunch."*—Aerobics instructor

Whether you are a weekend warrior, a fitness buff, or a serious athlete, it can be a challenge trying to squeeze in time to eat. You are likely juggling some combination of training, work, school, and sleep, plus the task of trying to fuel your body for sport activities. If your sport or fitness activity takes you on the road, you have the additional challenge of choosing foods for optimal performance from a restaurant or fast-food place.

When I was competing on the track and cross-country teams in college, I would wind up in the team doctor's office every year to "rule out mononucleosis." I was chronically tired, but no medical condition could explain my fatigue. Looking back at my lifestyle, I have no doubt that my problem stemmed from eating too little and getting too little sleep. I would eat only a minimal breakfast because I needed the time for my extra morning run. I'd cycle to school. Then I normally skipped lunch because it interfered with my afternoon training. By the end of the day, I was literally running on empty. (I was a physical education major back then and not yet nutritionally enlightened.)

Depending on your sport, be it a recreational or serious endeavor, and how long you train, you may need several thousand calories a day. To meet these energy needs, you must both eat an adequate amount of food and be mindful of the types of food to eat. Otherwise, training and performance are likely to suffer.

CREATING A FOOD FOUNDATION

Although popular diet books spurn carbohydrates, this nutrient is incredibly vital for fueling muscles—especially for endurance events. Carbohydrates are such an important fuel for exercise that muscles have a special form for storing them, called glycogen. Unlike the glycogen in the liver, which helps maintain a steady blood sugar level, muscle glycogen is used exclusively for fueling activity. Even if your blood sugar is low, muscle will not part with its precious glycogen reserve. This is because muscles need to have energy available at all times to be prepared for the fight-or-flight response during times of danger. Just as you need to keep gas in your car because you can't take off without it, so must your muscles start off with an optimal amount of glycogen fuel in the tank.

Numerous studies have shown that when muscle glycogen stores are emptied, exhaustion sets in. An average of 90 minutes of continuous aerobic exercise drains these vital energy stores. This critical point of depletion is also known as "hitting the wall."

Glycogen stores need to be replenished daily. If you are training daily and are not eating enough carbohydrates, you may feel chronically tired or just not up to your training. There may also be psychological consequences. You may begin to doubt your abilities, or worse, you may think that you need to train longer, which would deplete your glycogen stores even further and make you even more exhausted.

The 6-5-4-3-2 nutrition countdown serves as a good baseline food foundation (see chapter 1). But if you are training for an hour or more each day, you need a more powerful foundation in the form of *additional* carbohydrates to replenish what you have lost. Study after study has demonstrated the importance of eating an adequate amount of carbohydrates to prevent exhaustion, enhance training, and increase performance. Table 11.1 shows how important carbohydrates are to various forms of exercise.

TABLE 11.1 ESTIMATED CARBOHYDRATE NEEDS FOR SPORTS

Activity	Estimated calories used		Carbs burned (g)	Carb food equivalent (slices of bread)
	Calories/ minute	Total calories		
Running				
2 miles	20	215	50-55	3
10 km	18	700	150-170	10-11
26.2 miles (marathon)	15	2,800	500-550	33-37
Swimming (front crawl)				
200 m	25	50	12-15	1
1,500 m	20	400	90-100	6-7
Cycling				
1 hr	17	1,020	230-250	15-17

Data for a 70-kg (approximately 150-lb.) individual.

Adapted from "Carbohydrates for Exercise: Dietary Demands for Optimal Performance" by D.L. Costill, *International Journal of Sports Medicine*, 1988; 9:5. With permission of Georg Thieme Verlag.

If you are training over 60 minutes a day, you need to get at least 50 to 60 percent of your calories from carbohydrates, depending on your energy needs. Technically, you need 6 to 10 grams of carbohydrates per kilogram of weight, depending on how long you train. For someone weighing 70 kilograms (roughly 150 pounds), this amounts to 420 to 700 grams of carbohydrates.

To get an idea of how many carbohydrates are in certain foods, check out the Nutrition Facts on the food label. In the meanwhile, here are the general amounts of carbohydrates per food group:

Food group	Carbohydrates (g) per serving
Grains	15
Fruit	15
Dairy	12
Vegetables	5

For many endurance athletes or fitness enthusiasts, this means eating at least nine servings of grains and eight servings of fruits to meet their increased carbohydrate needs. This may sound like a huge amount of food. It's not. For example, one cup of hot cereal is equal to two grain servings. Most athletes can easily eat four pancakes, which is equivalent to four servings from the grain group. One bagel is about three servings from the grain group. Your food foundation supports your training and ultimately your performance. Ironically, many athletes neglect their diets until a competition is upon them. You can't suddenly begin working out one week prior to the main event. Similarly, nutrition needs to be consistent over the long haul—not just right before competition.

Quality Carbohydrates

The type of carbohydrate can also make a difference to performance, especially in endurance activities. Carbohydrates that enter the bloodstream at a slow, steady rate are beneficial to eat before performance. This type of carbohydrate has a low glycemic index. The glycemic index is a number that reflects how a specific food affects blood sugar levels. Low-glycemic-index foods are the best to eat before workouts or competition because they are released more slowly and result in steadier, more sustained blood sugar levels. See table 11.2 for the glycemic index of various foods.

The glycemic index is affected by many factors, including the presence of fiber and fat. Even how the food was cooked can be a factor. Keep in mind that the glycemic index is not a way to determine if foods are particularly healthy. For example, ice cream has a low glycemic index because of its high fat content, but I would not recommend eating it before a workout! Also, eating different foods together (as in a meal) gives an entirely different glycemic index number for each food. Overall, the best-quality carbohydrates

TABLE 11.2 GLYCEMIC INDEX OF COMMON FOODS

Food	Glycemic index	Food	Glycemic index
Waffles	76	Apple	38
Apple juice, unsweetened	40	Apricots, dried	31
Cranberry juice cocktail (Ocean Spray)	68	Banana, ripe	51
Orange juice	50	Banana, underripe	42
Gatorade	78	Cherries, raw	22
Bagel, white (Lender's)	72	Dates, dried	103
Cracked wheat bread	53	Fruit cocktail, canned	55
White bread	70	Grapes	46
All-Bran cereal (Kellogg's)	42	Kiwi	53
Bran Buds cereal (Kellogg's)	58	Mango	51
Coco Pops (Kellogg's)	77	Orange	31
Corn Chex (Nabisco)	83	Peach, raw	42
Corn Flakes (Kellogg's)	81	Peaches, canned in natural juice	38
Cream of Wheat (Nabisco)	66	Pear	38
Cream of Wheat, instant (Nabisco)	74	Pineapple	59
Grape-Nuts (Post)	71	Raisins	64
Life cereal (Quaker)	66	Baked beans	48
Oat bran	55	Chickpeas (garbanzo beans)	28
Oats, instant	66	Kidney beans	28
Raisin Bran (Kellogg's)	61	Lentils	29
Rice Krispies (Kellogg's)	82	Pinto beans, canned	45
Shredded Wheat	75	Ensure bar, chocolate	43
Barley	25	Ensure Plus, vanilla	40
White rice, long grain	56	Macaroni	48
Brown rice	55	Spaghetti	38
Puffed rice cakes	78	Power Bar, chocolate	56
Rye crispbread	64	Ironman PR bar, chocolate	39
Milk, skim	32	Potato, baked	85
Milk, low-fat chocolate	34	Sweet potato	61
Yogurt, low-fat	31	Carrots	47

Adapted from Foster-Powell et al. (2002).

in a training diet are unrefined and high in fiber (such as whole wheat bread rather than white bread).

PREEXERCISE MEAL

What, how much, and when should you eat prior to competition? What about on a day-to-day basis for routine workouts? *When* you eat your meals and snacks can significantly affect your performance both in competition and in routine training. Your stomach should not be full of food. Otherwise, you could feel uncomfortable or nauseated (or even vomit), partly because your exercising muscles must compete with your stomach for the blood supply. The more intensely you exercise (for instance, sprinting rather than slow jogging), the more intensely your muscles need blood.

At rest, about 25 percent of normal blood flow goes to the digestive tract. During hard exercise, however, only 4 percent of the blood flow is delivered to the gastrointestinal (GI) system, and 85 percent is supplied to the muscle. Large meals increase blood flow to the GI tract, diverting it from exercising muscle. After a meal, food typically empties from your stomach in about three to four hours. Ideally, you should eat a meal about three to four hours before working out. You can eat one to two hours prior to exercise—just eat less food. When you eat should determine the composition and size of the meal (or snack, if it's close to workout time).

Carbohydrates are the nutrients digested most quickly. Foods containing protein take a little longer to break down. Fat packs a double digestive whammy: it takes the longest to digest, and the presence of fat in the stomach slows down the entire rate of digestion. Aim for high-carbohydrate and low-fat foods before you train or compete. In general, a meal needs to be large enough to avert hunger and provide energy, yet not so large that it causes gastric distress. Here's an example of a high-carbohydrate meal:

1 cup nonfat milk

1 turkey sandwich (2 ounces turkey, 2 slices whole wheat bread)

1 cup applesauce

2 graham crackers

This meal has 92 grams of carbohydrates and 515 calories, 70 percent of which are carbohydrate calories.

There will be occasions when you don't have the luxury of eating three to four hours before working out. It is still okay to eat, but you need to decrease the quantity of food proportionately (remember, you want an empty stomach for exercise). Here is a guideline to determine how many carbohydrates serious endurance athletes should eat, based on the time before competition or workout:

Time before training or competition	Eat this amount of carbohydrate per kg of weight
1 hr	1 g
2 hr	2 g
3 hr	3 g
4 hr	4 g

Keep in mind your individual tolerance to food and timing of exercise. You need to experiment to find out what feels good to eat before and during exercise.

CARBOHYDRATE LOADING

If you participate in an aerobic sport lasting 90 minutes or longer, such as cycling, soccer, marathons, and triathlons, you can benefit from a scientifically validated eating protocol called carbohydrate loading. It's helpful to understand why this type of eating is beneficial.

Study after study has shown that when muscle glycogen stores are emptied by endurance events lasting 90 minutes or longer, exhaustion sets in. Even elite endurance athletes have difficulty training when their carbohydrate intake is inadequate. Therefore, athletes who train 90 minutes or longer regularly can benefit from carbohydrate loading. Keeping day-to-day glycogen stores full is important to support the demands of long training.

Carbohydrate loading is both a training and an eating regimen that increases carbohydrate stores to their optimal capacity. Endurance training increases the storage capacity for glycogen (like having a 20-gallon gas tank rather than a 15-gallon one), and carbohydrates are what fill it. The protocol begins six days before competition by gradually tapering down training from 90 minutes per day to no training. This tapering is accompanied by three days of a regular training diet (a minimum of 50 percent of calories from carbohydrate) followed by three days of a high-carbohydrate diet (70 percent carbohydrate calories). See table 11.3.

A general rule to ensure optimal carbohydrate intake is to aim for about 600 grams of carbohydrates per day. But to figure out your specific needs, use this formula: 10 grams of carbohydrates for every kilogram you weigh (2.2 pounds = 1 kilogram). For example, if you weigh 125 pounds, you should aim for 568 grams of carbohydrates per day.

$$(125 \text{ pounds}/2.2) \times 10 = 568$$

Despite the implication of the term *loading,* this protocol is not about overeating but rather increasing the proportion of carbohydrates in your diet while tapering your training.

Carbohydrates During Exercise

For events lasting 60 minutes or longer, there is no doubt that consuming carbohydrates during the activity improves performance. You need about

TABLE 11.3 CARBOHYDRATE-LOADING PROTOCOL

Days before competition	Training before competition	Diet
6	90 minutes	50% carbs
5	40 minutes	50% carbs
4	40 minutes	50% carbs
3	20 minutes	70% carbs
2	20 minutes	70% carbs
1	Rest	70% carbs
0	Competition	

From "Carbohydrates, Muscle Glycogen, and Muscle Glycogen Supercompensation" by W. Sherman, 1983. In Ergogenic Aids in Sport (p. 13) by M.H. Williams (ed.), Champaign, IL: Human Kinetics. Copyright 1983 by M.H. Williams. Adapted by permission.

30 to 60 grams of carbohydrates per hour of activity. This is easily found in sports drinks containing 4 percent to 8 percent carbohydrates. Sports gels or solid food can work too, as long as an adequate amount of fluids are also consumed (discussed later in this chapter). Even if you exercise less than one hour, a carbohydrate-containing sports drink is beneficial, especially if you work out in the morning on an empty stomach.

Carbohydrates After Exercise

Carbohydrates are equally as important for recovery immediately after endurance exercise and during the following two hours. This is when glycogen stores are built back up most quickly. While low-glycemic-index foods are helpful before exercise, high-glycemic-index foods are helpful after exercise to help refuel muscles. Table 11.4 gives guidelines for keeping those carbohydrates adequate to fuel fitness.

TABLE 11.4 PERFORMANCE CARBOHYDRATES BY THE NUMBERS

Carbs needed	When
6-10 g/kg of weight	Training
30-60 g/hr	During exercise
1.5 g/kg of weight	During the first 30 minutes after 90 minutes of exercise and again every 2 hr for 4 to 6 hr
10 g/kg of weight	Carbohydrate loading (before endurance events lasting 90 minutes or longer)

ROAD WARRIORS

Traveling can be a challenge for any athlete, from the college athlete who gets "meal money" for the first time to the experienced competitor at an out-of-town triathlon. In previous chapters, I discussed the challenges of eating on the road, but athletes face another problem: getting enough carbohydrates. Ironically, in your quest for the low-fat-food grail, you may end up with foods that are too low in calories and carbohydrates (high-octane fuel for the muscles). For example, McDonald's grilled chicken Caesar salad with fat-free herb vinaigrette dressing is low in fat, but it is also devoid of carbohydrates. Here are some guidelines for eating while traveling:

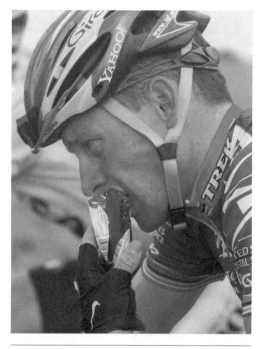

Energy bars can be a good way to refuel your body during intense exercise.

- Order low-fat foods.
- Order extra carbohydrates (such as a baked potato, cereal, rice, low-fat muffin, or juice).
- Stash extra carbohydrates, such as energy bars or dried fruit, for times when you're stuck at an airport or a competition goes on longer than planned and you are caught without food. Table 11.5 lists some specific best bets for traveling athletes. This is just a representative guide; there are many combinations and ways to order heavy on the carbs.

PUMPING PROTEIN

The Institute of Medicine's 2002 DRI report on protein and physical activity concluded that there is a lack of compelling evidence that healthy adults undertaking resistance or endurance exercise need more protein. However, the American College of Sports Medicine recommends increased protein for endurance and strength-training athletes (see also table 11.6).

1.2 to 1.4 g/kg for endurance athletes

1.6 to 1.7 g/kg for strength-training athletes

Both organizations, however, agree that these needs can be met through diet alone. Chances are that you're getting more than enough protein to

TABLE 11.5 ORDERING FAST FOODS HEAVY ON THE CARBS

Food	Calories	Carbs (g)
Burger King		
BK Veggie Burger	330	45
Chicken Caesar salad with croutons and		
light Italian dressing	300	23
Orange juice	<u>140</u>	<u>33</u>
	770	101 (52%)
Carl's Jr.		
Charbroiled BBQ Chicken sandwich	290	41
Plain baked potato	<u>290</u>	<u>68</u>
	580	109 (75%)
Jack in the Box		
Chicken Fajita Pita	330	35
10-oz. orange juice	<u>140</u>	<u>32</u>
	470	67 (57%)
McDonald's		
Fruit 'n Yogurt Parfait	380	53
Low-fat apple bran muffin	<u>300</u>	<u>61</u>
	680	114 (67%)
Subway		
12" Honey mustard turkey sandwich with		
cucumbers	550	90 (65%)
Taco Bell		
2 Chicken Fiesta Burritos	740	96 (52%)
Wendy's		
Plain baked potato	310	72
Chili, large	<u>300</u>	<u>31</u>
	610	103 (68%)

These meals range from 470 to 770 calories but can be easily adjusted to meet your energy needs. All provide at least 50% of their calories from carbohydrates.

TABLE 11.6 PROTEIN BY THE NUMBERS

	Protein (g/kg of weight)	Protein for a 70-kg (150-lb.) person
DRI	0.8 g	56 g
Endurance athletes	1.2-1.4 g	84-98 g
Strength-training athletes	1.6-1.7 g	112-119 g

support new muscle growth. Muscle is made up of 22 percent protein and 70 percent water. Therefore, one pound of muscle contains only 3 1/2 ounces of protein.

To add one pound of pure muscle in a week, the body needs an additional 10 to 14 grams of protein a day (that's about 12 ounces of milk or half a chicken breast). The body can add only two pounds of muscle in a week. But protein alone does not build muscle. It takes strength training and additional calories.

Endurance athletes benefit from additional protein because when carbohydrate stores are depleted, the body turns to muscle as a fuel. When you're out of carbohydrates, your body burns up the indispensable branched-chain amino acids (leucine, isoleucine, and valine) from muscle. In fact, when a healthy person becomes chronically ill, the largest single contributor to protein loss is muscle. Carbohydrates spare muscle from being broken down as an energy source.

FLUIDS AND SPORTS DRINKS

Water is the nutrient that athletes neglect the most. This forgotten nutrient is essential to life and to performance. It is so abundant, inexpensive, and readily available that it is frequently taken for granted.

There is no doubt that dehydration decreases exercise performance. Loss of water from the body of as little as 2 percent of body weight can significantly impair performance. Yet without making a conscious effort to drink water, you can suffer fluid deficits amounting to 3 percent of body weight before you feel thirsty.

By the time you do feel thirsty, dehydration has most likely set in, partly because the thirst response is blunted during physical exercise. Additionally, many studies have shown that athletes do not drink enough to replace the water lost, even when given the opportunity. Here are drinking guidelines to keep your body optimally hydrated:

- **Before exercise:** Two hours before exercise, drink 14 to 22 ounces of water.
- **During exercise:** At the start of exercise, drink 6 to 12 ounces every 15 to 20 minutes.
- **After exercise:** Drink from one to one and a half times the amount you've lost in sweat.

To figure out how much water weight you've lost through sweating, you need to monitor your weight. Two cups of water weigh one pound. Therefore, you need to replace every pound of sweat lost with at least two cups of water. For example, if you weighed 150 pounds before a workout and 148 pounds after, you need to drink four cups of water to replace your fluid deficit.

What's Best to Drink: Water or Sports Drinks?

Plain water generally works if you are working out for less than an hour. But drinks containing 4 to 8 percent carbohydrates work better if you are working out intensely for one hour or longer. Sodium and other electrolytes offer little advantage during exercise lasting less than three to four hours, but sodium is helpful after exercise for two reasons:

1. Sodium keeps the fluid you drink in your body longer (rather than being excreted).

2. Keeping blood sodium levels at an even keel helps increase the desire to drink.

Most sports drinks do not contain enough sodium for this purpose. But it's easy to eat some high-sodium foods, such as soup, popcorn, and pretzels, along with fluids after a workout. This extra salt is recommended mainly for serious athletes engaged in heavy training.

ERGOGENIC AIDS

Many athletes and fitness enthusiasts have searched for a magic pill or supplement that offers that extra edge of reduced recovery time or increased energy or strength. These "miracle" substances are referred to as ergogenic aids. By definition, an ergogenic aid is something that can increase the ability to do work.

During my competitive running days before I was in the nutrition field, I tried all kinds of nutritional ergogenic aids. I once had a well-meaning coach tell me that I should eat enough wheat germ that if I were cut, I'd bleed wheat germ. Fortunately, wheat germ is a food, and no harm came from eating so much of it.

Many of the products sold to increase performance, such as bee pollen, are useless. Why are they sold? Money. Many of the claims for ergogenic aids are made by the companies that sell them. This multimillion-dollar industry has a lot to gain by preying on the desires of athletes to gain the competitive edge.

Some athletes and fitness buffs truly believe a particular supplement works. In fact, sometimes an athlete believes so strongly in a supplement that any inert substance, such as a sugar pill, will work. This is known as the placebo effect, or the power of belief. The performance benefit results from this placebo phenomenon, not from the actual supplement. Author and researcher Dan Benardot of the Laboratory for Elite Athlete Performance at

Georgia State University described such a phenomenon. He was conducting a test of the supplement creatine to see if it could improve performance. Neither researcher nor athletes knew who was getting a placebo and who was getting creatine (a double-blind study). However, one particular athlete was absolutely certain she had the creatine pill and indeed improved her performance. It turned out, however, that she had taken the placebo pill. But her belief was powerful enough to improve her performance!

Sometimes a coincidence leads athletes to believe that a nutritional aid works. For example, if an athlete breaks a record on the same day that he or she took bee pollen, it is easy to attribute the outstanding performance to the supplement. The success probably resulted instead from hard training and other factors.

It can be difficult to evaluate the claims of ergogenic aids because the benefits are established using pseudoscience at best. Here are a few pointers for evaluating products that claim to help performance.

- Remember that no supplement or ergogenic aid can replace training, a healthy diet, and adequate sleep.
- If it sounds too good to be true, it probably is.
- Is the product safe? Who says?
- Is the claim consistent with good research and your particular sport or activity?
- What is the motivation behind the claim?
- How is the supplement marketed?
- Are the ingredients effective?

Some popular ergogenic aids are reviewed in table 11.7.

TABLE 11.7 POPULAR ERGOGENIC AIDS

Supplement	Claim	Demonstrated benefits	Possible side effects
Amino acids: arginine, lysine, and ornithine	• Increase muscle • Decrease fat • Increase growth hormone	No	1. Metabolic imbalance from single amino acids 2. Gastrointestinal (GI) distress
Branched-chain amino acids	• Prevent fatigue • Improve endurance	Equivocal	1. Decrease water absorption if taken during exercise. 2. GI distress
Caffeine	• Improves endurance	Yes 3-13 mg/kg 1 hr before exercise	1. Rapid pulse 2. GI distress 3. Diarrhea 4. Nausea 5. Doses of 9-13 mg/kg can raise blood caffeine to illegal levels for NCAA and Olympic competition.
Carnitine (L-carnitine)	• Improves endurance • Increases fat burning for fuel	No	1. Increased frequency and severity of seizures in those who have a history of seizures 2. D-carnitine can cause carnitine deficiency. 3. DL-carnitine has been associated with myasthenia syndrome, including severe weakness and muscle wasting.
Chromium picolinate	• Increases muscle • Decreases fat	No FTC ordered 3 of the largest distributors to stop making these unsubstantiated claims	1. Safe at adequate intake levels, 20-35 µg depending on age and sex 2. Case of rhabdomyolysis (muscle cell injury) reported at 1,200 µg/day

(continued)

TABLE 11.7 *(continued)*

Supplement	Claim	Demonstrated benefits	Possible side effects
Creatine	• Increases muscle • Improves performance of brief, high-intensity activities	Mostly yes 20-25 g/day for 5 to 7 days; 5 g/day thereafter	1. No long-term safety data 2. May stress liver and kidneys
Glutamine or L-glutamic acid	• Improves immunity • Prevents overtraining syndrome	Equivocal	1. May induce mania in people with bipolar disorder
Glycerol	• Improves fluid balance • Improves endurance	Equivocal	1. Bloating 2. Nausea 3. Vomiting 4. Headache 5. Contraindicated for those with diabetes, high blood pressure, or kidney disorders
HMB (beta-hydroxy-beta-methyl-butyrate)	• Increases muscle • Decreases fat • Increases strength and power	Equivocal	None reported
MCT (medium-chain triglycerides)	• Decrease fat • Improve endurance • Spare glycogen	Mostly no	1. GI distress 2. Nausea and vomiting 3. Irritability 4. Diarrhea
Pyruvate	• Weight loss • Improved endurance performance	Questionable yes	1. Diarrhea 2. Bloating 3. Gas
Whey protein	• Increases muscle	No	High doses may cause 1. Fatigue 2. Nausea 3. Cramps 4. Bloating

Source: Natural Medicine Database. Jellin JM, Gregory PJ, Batz F, Hitchens K et al. Pharmacist's Letter-Prescriber's Letter Natural Medicine Comprehensive Database, 4th ed, Therapeutic Research Faculty: Stockton, CA, 2002.

PART IV

Quick and Tasty Meals

CHAPTER 12

Cooking Secrets in a Snap

"Cook? What's that?"—Single real estate agent

Some of my clients are embarrassed to admit that they don't cook. I know few people who relish the thought of coming home and making dinner after putting in a full workday. I'm one of them—even though I've written three cookbooks! I do enjoy cooking on the weekends when the pace of our family life is more leisurely. For some people, even the thought of cooking makes them feel exhausted. But preparing dinner doesn't have to be a big production. Remember, you don't have to have hot-cooked meals to enjoy good nutrition. In this chapter, I share timesaving measures to get your meals prepared in a flash so you can have more time to enjoy your evening.

As you learned in chapter 1, successful eating on the run begins with planning. It's important to plan some meals ahead of time and to have the ingredients on hand, especially when you know you will be home for dinner. This alone saves gobs of time and spares you the aggravation of staring at the cupboards waiting for divine inspiration night after night. Just knowing there is a plan for a meal and the ingredients to support it also reduces a layer of stress. For example, I know a busy couple who both had very stressful jobs and long hours. When they got home, they were simply too pooped to cook, yet they were tired of eating out night after night. To their surprise, they found that knowing what was for dinner when they came home and having the ingredients to make it was much more relaxing. This planning took the dread out of the age-old question "What's for dinner?" and actually saved time compared with going out to eat.

This chapter focuses on the keys to get you out of the kitchen faster: organization, using already-prepped food, planned-overs, and timesaving gadgets.

BASIC ORGANIZATION

How would your rate your cupboards and refrigerator?

1. Disaster area
2. Organized mess
3. Creatures from the black lagoon
4. Mystery area (or, What's behind pantry door number 2?)
5. Room for improvement

Kitchen storage space seems to be a problem in most homes. Kitchen supplies expand to fill the storage space. If you increase storage space but fail to organize it, you could end up with a bigger mess. When you do not know where an item is, you waste valuable time hunting for it, and you may get frustrated by the search. The answer to avoiding these scavenger hunts lies in organization.

Following are some ideas for arranging kitchen storage areas. The basic principle is to group items that will be used together, similar to the way that grocery stores are arranged. Try implementing the ideas that will save you time.

Cupboards

1. Keep frequently used items within easy reach.
2. Alphabetize your spices for speedy identification. You'll be surprised at how much time that effort can save.
3. Store utensils and foods near the areas where you'll use them most (pot holders next to the oven, pans by the stove).
4. Store foods with the labels facing out so that you can easily identify them.
5. Group your foods for easy locating:
   - Bottled items
   - Canned items
   - Dry foods
   - Grains and beans
   - Packaged foods
   - Paper goods
6. Install a "step-up" shelf (a shelf that is half the usual width or less, placed between two other shelves) for small items such as cups, saucers, small dishes, and spices.
7. Store these bigger items in a separate storage area: appliances, gadgets, mixing bowls, pots, and pans.

Drawers

1. Eliminate any junk or clutter.
2. Partition drawers for organizing utensils: baking utensils, eating utensils, gadgets, knives, stove-top utensils.

Countertop

1. Keep these regularly used appliances ready to go on the counter:
   - Blender
   - Can opener
   - Food processor
   - Mixer
   - Toaster
2. Place these food staples in canisters on the counter to save time digging them out of drawers and cabinets:
   - Beans
   - Bread (in bread box)
   - Flour
   - Noodles
   - Rice
   - Other staples
3. Place grazing foods ready to go in a basket.
4. If feasible, hang gadgets, utensils, or pots on the wall closest to where you use them.

Refrigerator

1. Take advantage of built-in organizers such as the margarine keeper and vegetable drawer.
2. Store foods in easy-to-see containers such as jars and transparent dishes.
3. Keep frequently used items in spots that are easy to reach.
4. Divide your refrigerator space into fives areas for the following categories of foods: beverages, dairy, produce, proteins, leftovers.
5. Use the FIFO (first in, first out) system. This helps prevent wasted food and multiple containers of the same foods.

ADVANCE PREPARATION

Food preparation steps often seem like going back one step to move ahead two. Chopping, slicing, and dicing food can be time-consuming and boring. Such tasks often present the most obstacles when deciding what to eat.

The more rungs you eliminate on the food-preparation ladder, the more time you have to enjoy. Having food already prepped or ready to go when you need it is essential for grazers. Already-prepped food also makes it easier to throw together an evening meal when you feel drained after a hard day. This was made ever so clear to me when I began doing cooking demonstrations on television shows. My food was always prepped in advance. A meal that would normally take 15 to 30 minutes literally was reduced to less than 5 minutes on camera! Most people don't have cooking assistants at their disposal, but the ideas below can save oodles of time (also check out figure 12.1).

PRE-PREPPED FOODS AT THE GROCERY STORE

Canned
(preferably no added salt)

Beans

Black

Garbanzo

Kidney

Pinto

Baked beans, vegetarian

Refried beans, fat-free

Soups

Dairy
(fat-free and low-fat varieties)

Cheeses

Shredded

Single-serving size

Meats

Boneless, skinless chicken

Chicken breast tidbits

Chicken, fully cooked
    rotisserie-style

Ground turkey breast

Turkey breast medallions,
    tenderloins, cutlets

Produce

Cabbage, shredded

Carrots, baby

Carrots, sliced or shredded

Cherry or grape tomatoes
    (rather than whole tomatoes)

Lettuce, shredded

Mushrooms, sliced

Onions, chopped

Salad bags, assorted

Spinach, chopped

Frozen

Berries, unsweetened (raspberries,
    mixed berries, blueberries)

Peppers, chopped

Onions, chopped

Mushrooms, sliced

Figure 12.1 There are a variety of nutritious pre-prepped selections available.

Buy It Already-Prepped

Instead of slicing and dicing your knuckles to the bone, consider buying your food in the least time-consuming form. I can think of no better example than grated cheese, which is available in reduced-fat varieties. Not only do you save prep time, but you don't have to clean the grater.

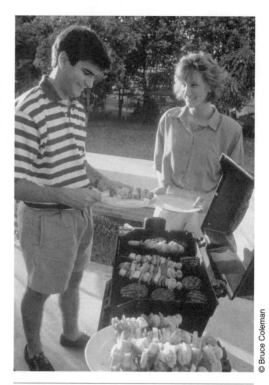

For a 10-minute, tasty meal, grill precut veggies and meat marinaded the night before.

You can buy turkey in many ready-to-cook varieties: sliced, tidbits, cutlets, and ground, not to mention already-cooked turkey and chicken strips. Packaged fresh gourmet-style salads, baby carrots, and assorted chopped vegetables are available in the produce section washed and ready to eat. The only disadvantage of buying food already prepped is the added cost. I think it's worth it. You may actually save money when you consider what your time is worth or the amount you spend on take-out food, which costs considerably more.

Pre-prep Food Yourself

Prepping food yourself is a good option, especially if you are watching your budget. The best technique is to prepare all the food at one time in advance, which saves you time in the long run and makes the food readily available when you need it. A food processor saves you even more time. Otherwise, a good, sharp knife will do.

Ready, set, go. Set aside a time for batch chopping, slicing, and dicing. Consider doing it right after grocery shopping, before you put your food away. Next, use the Baggie method of food control: divide bulk items such as vegetables into smaller batches in plastic bags for convenient storage and easy access. Clear storage bowls also do the trick. With everything sliced and ready to go, you can put together a meal in a hurry.

PLANNED LEFTOVERS

Planned-overs are intentional leftovers. With this technique, also known as batch cooking, you take advantage of your cooking moments. When you have time to cook, double or even triple your favorite recipe. By doing this, you can prepare multiple meals in nearly the same amount of time as it takes to fix one. Then you have an instant home-cooked meal ready to eat in a jiffy, usually just a zap away.

Making planned-overs can be as simple as cooking a few extra chicken breasts or meats and freezing them for later. Here's how to make the most of planned-overs:

1. Divide your meals into individual freezer containers to make your own frozen dinners. This method helps preserve nutrients because you won't reheat the same batch of food over and over.

2. Store meals in containers in which they can be reheated. If you use a microwave, be sure your container is microwave-proof.

3. Rotate your planned-overs to keep them from becoming boring.

4. Label and date your planned-overs, or else it is easy to forget what's in a container and when it was made.

5. For a cook-free workweek with homestyle food, make a week's worth of meals ahead on the weekend.

TIMESAVING GADGETS

Here are a few gadgets worth investing in. Of course, gadgets save time only if you use them; otherwise, they can become just clutter. Pick and choose what can help you.

▰ Apple slicer/corer. This handy device cores and slices apples into even wedges. It's an inexpensive gadget that saves a lot of time.

▰ Cordless mixer. It's always ready to go when mounted on the wall with all of its attachments. There's no hassle searching for a mixer, and you are not confined to using it near an electric outlet. The only disadvantage is cordless mixers are not as powerful as traditional stand mixers.

▰ Crock-Pot. The nice thing about Crock-Pots is that you just throw together a few choice ingredients, set the thermostat, and off to work (or wherever) you go. You arrive home to a hot cooked meal without slaving over a hot stove. Some all-in-one meals that work well with Crock-Pots are stewed chicken, soups, and bean dishes (such as split peas, lentils, black beans, and chili).

▰ Garlic press. If you love fresh garlic flavor, a garlic press is the fastest way to get minced garlic. One squish through this little press and you have minced garlic, without the traditional tedious chopping.

▰ "Insta-hot" hot-water dispenser. This near-boiling water spigot resembles a built-in soap dispenser. Frankly, I never realized the timesaving value of this gadget until I received one as a gift. If you have used one at the water cooler at work, then you know how fast you can make tea and instant bean soups. I also use it to get a head start on boiling water for steaming vegetables or making pasta.

◢ Kitchen shears. Since I finally broke down and bought a pair, I don't how I survived without them. They have really simplified irksome tasks such as snipping parsley and chives. Many food packages also need to be cut open, and kitchen scissors do a quick job.

◢ Food processor. Don't tell me: you received one for a Christmas or wedding gift but still haven't gotten around to using it. The solution is to keep it on your counter ready to go with attachments nearby. It will save a lot of time.

◢ Immersible hand blender. This electric gadget is a speedy solution for mixing soups and sauces without all the cleanup of a traditional blender.

◢ Microwave. I don't need to extol this common kitchen item. Keep in mind that besides heating frozen meals and leftovers, a microwave can be used for full cooking, such as "baking" a potato. Microwave cooking preserves more nutrients than traditional cooking. One of the things I like best about microwave cooking is that it usually means fewer to dishes to clean.

Ten Timesaving Habits

If you adopt the practices listed here, your tour of duty in the kitchen will be much shorter.

1. Assemble all the ingredients, utensils, and pans before you begin cooking. This allows efficient cooking without having to stop and search.

2. To keep dishes to a minimum (and save time cleaning them), mix everything in a large measuring cup instead of a mixing bowl. Stir ingredients with a measuring spoon instead of a big spoon and use cooking and baking dishes that can double as serving dishes.

3. Make use of your downtime. For example, set the table while waiting for the microwave.

4. Keep track of foods and other essentials that need to be replaced so that you don't have to run to the store unexpectedly. Keep a pad and pen or an erasable board in your kitchen near the cupboards.

5. Serve buffet-style (everyone assembles their own plate). Meals such as turkey tacos, deli night, or a homestyle salad bar work well.

6. For easy vegetables, keep baby carrots or bagged salads in stock.

7. Try fresh pasta (from the deli section) rather than dried. It saves considerable cooking time. The quickest to fix is angel hair pasta. It takes only 60 seconds in boiling water.

8. Stockpile staples. Make sure you have an ample supply of routinely used food items.

9. Take advantage of one-dish meals (such as casseroles or rice bowls) and the 60-second meals in the next chapter.

10. Plan, plan, plan.

QUICK AND EASY MEALS

Here are some recipes for quick, easy, and nutritional meals to prepare if you're on the go. Special notes for vegans (vegetarians who eat no animal or dairy products) are included as designated by an asterisk.

1-2-3 Rotisserie Chicken

You get three different easy meals from one chicken—and you don't even have to cook the chicken!

Meal 1:

Buy a whole rotisserie-style chicken from your local grocery store or take-out place. Round out the chicken with your favorite vegetables and some baked beans. Be sure to reserve some leftover chicken to make the next two meals.

Meal 2:

You'll need barbecue sauce, ready-made pizza crust, and light mozzarella cheese. Toss about 1/2 cup of barbecue sauce with leftover chicken, then scatter it across the pizza crust. Sprinkle with 2 cups shredded mozzarella cheese. Bake at 350°F until bubbly. For extra flavor, garnish the pizza with a little red onion and chopped cilantro.

Meal 3:

Add leftover chicken to your favorite bagged salad. Toss in canned beans (such as kidney beans or garbanzo beans). Sprinkle with slivered almonds or walnut halves and toss with your favorite light dressing.

Quick Marinara Sauce with Angel Hair Pasta (serves 4)

This easy sauce is loaded with vitamin A thanks to the shredded carrot. One serving provides nearly 70 percent of your vitamin A needs for the day.

olive oil nonstick spray

chopped garlic (2 fresh cloves or 2 teaspoons from jar)

1 teaspoon dried oregano, crushed

1/4 teaspoon dried basil

1 carrot, finely grated

28-oz. can chopped stewed tomatoes

1/2 6-oz. can tomato paste

9-oz. package fresh angel hair pasta, cooked

4 tablespoons shredded deli-style Parmesan cheese

Nutrition:	
291 calories	14 g protein
55 g carbs	4 g fat
1 g sat. fat	5 g cholesterol
1,012 mg sodium	6 g fiber

Spray a large nonstick skillet with nonstick cooking spray. Add garlic, oregano, basil, and carrots. Cook and stir over medium-high heat for 2 minutes. Add stewed tomatoes and tomato paste. Cook until bubbly. Pour over pasta. Top with Parmesan cheese.

Timesaving Tip: Double the sauce, toss half with the hot pasta, and freeze the rest for a future meal.

*To make this vegan, simply omit the Parmesan cheese.

Spinach Cheese Pasta (serves 4)

When vegetables are already an integral part of a dish, they're easy to get into your diet.

olive oil nonstick spray

chopped garlic (2 fresh cloves or 2 teaspoons from jar)

10-oz. package frozen chopped spinach, thawed and well drained

1 cup nonfat cottage cheese

1/2 cup shredded deli-style Parmesan cheese

9-oz. package fresh angel hair pasta, cooked

Nutrition:

298 calories	23 g protein
41 g carbs	5 g fat
2 g sat. fat	15 g cholesterol
687 mg sodium	3 g fiber

Spray a large nonstick skillet with nonstick cooking spray. Add garlic and cook over medium-high heat until fragrant, about 1 minute. Add spinach and stir. Add cheeses and stir thoroughly until cheese is melted. Toss in pasta.

Timesaving Tip: To quickly thaw spinach, heat in microwave, or place frozen spinach in the refrigerator to thaw before you go to work in the morning.

*To make this vegan, replace the cottage cheese with crumbled tofu, and use soy cheese instead of the Parmesan cheese.

Turkey Chili (serves 8)

This high-fiber meal tastes so good as leftovers!

1 lb. ground turkey breast

1/2 cup chopped onion (medium whole onion or precut and packaged from produce section)

3 16-oz. cans pinto or kidney beans

28-oz. can chopped stewed tomatoes

1 tablespoon chili powder

1 tablespoon cumin powder

1/2 cup salsa

1/2 cup grated light cheddar cheese

Nutrition:

285 calories	29 g protein
33 g carbs	5 g fat
2 g sat. fat	38 g cholesterol
899 mg sodium	12 g fiber

In a 4-quart pot, cook the turkey and onions, stirring until the turkey is no longer pink. Add beans, tomatoes, seasonings, and salsa. Cook until heated through. If desired, garnish with cheese.

Timesaving Tip: Open cans while turkey is cooking. Buy precut onions either frozen or fresh.

*To make this vegan, omit the turkey breast and cheddar cheese.

Relax-While-It-Cooks Foil Chicken (serves 4)

Keeping the skin on the potato not only saves time, but it increases the fiber value.

1 cup barbecue sauce

4 skinless, boneless chicken breasts

1 red or green bell pepper, sliced

2 carrots, diagonally cut

2 small potatoes, washed and thinly sliced

Nutrition:	
260 calories	29 g protein
24 g carbs	4 g fat
1 g sat. fat	73 g cholesterol
589 mg sodium	3 g fiber

Preheat the oven to 350°F. Line a baking sheet with foil. Place half the barbecue sauce on the foil. Top with chicken. Pour remaining sauce over chicken. Add the cut vegetables. Add another layer of foil, and fold the four sides together. Bake about 40 minutes, until chicken is no longer pink when cut in the center.

Timesaving Tip: Make additional chicken breasts for a next-day barbecue sandwich or barbecue chicken pizza. Don't worry about exact measurements—the eyeball technique works just fine here.

Tostadas (makes 6 tostadas)

6 corn tortillas

16-oz. can fat-free vegetarian refried beans

1 1/2 cups shredded lettuce

2 tomatoes, chopped

1 cup shredded light cheddar cheese

salsa

Nutrition (1 tostada):	
184 calories	12 g protein
27 g carbs	4 g fat
2 g sat. fat	14 g cholesterol
538 mg sodium	6 g fiber

Preheat the oven to 350°F. Place corn tortillas on a baking sheet, and spray the tortillas with nonstick spray. Bake until light brown (about 7 minutes). Layer the remaining ingredients on the tortillas in the following order (or as you like): beans, lettuce, tomatoes, cheese, and salsa.

Timesaving Tips: You can buy shredded lettuce in the produce section. While tortillas are crisping in the oven, prepare garnishes. Have everyone assemble their own tostada to suit their taste and save time.

*To make this vegan, eliminate the cheddar cheese.

Oregano Chicken Soup (serves 6)

Freeze extra bowls of this soup and you are only minutes away from a satisfying meal. Serve with a whole wheat roll and a glass of low-fat milk.

6 cups reduced-salt chicken broth

2 teaspoons oregano

1/2 teaspoon celery seed

1/2 cup chopped onion

3 skinless, boneless chicken breasts

28-oz. can chopped stewed tomatoes (including juice)

2 carrots, sliced

1 cup dark green leafy vegetables, chopped

Nutrition:	
154 calories	19 g protein
15 g carbs	4 g fat
1 g sat. fat	42 g cholesterol
495 mg sodium	4 g fiber

In a 4-quart pot, combine all ingredients. Bring to a boil. Reduce heat and cover with a lid. Cook until chicken is cooked through and pink tinge is gone in center (about 30 minutes). Remove chicken. Cut or shred it into bite-size pieces. Place chicken pieces back in pot. Soup's ready!

Timesaving Tip: You can buy fresh chopped spinach and onions in the produce section.

Make-Ahead Stuffed Potatoes

This is a family favorite that gets a quicker start in the microwave.

4 medium potatoes, washed

16-oz. fat-free cottage cheese

1 cup shredded light cheddar cheese

Nutrition (2 halves):	
274 calories	27 g protein
30 g carbs	5 g fat
4 g sat. fat	30 g cholesterol
599 mg sodium	2 g fiber

Pierce the potatoes with a fork. Microwave 12 to 16 minutes, rotating the potatoes every 3 to 4 minutes for more even cooking. Cut potatoes in half. Scoop out the potato pulp, leaving a thin layer of the skin. In a large bowl, combine the potato pulp, cottage cheese, and half the shredded cheese. With a mixer, blend until thoroughly combined. Fill the potato shells with the potato mixture. Top with the remaining shredded cheese. Broil in a conventional oven until the cheese is melted.

Timesaving Tip: Make ahead and freeze. Eat for breakfast, lunch, snack, or dinner.

Fajitas (serves 4)

2 tablespoons fat-free Italian dressing

1 tablespoon lime or lemon juice

1 medium onion, sliced into thin
strips

2 medium bell peppers (red, yellow,
or green), sliced into thin strips

1 lb. lean meat, chopped (turkey,
chicken, or round steak)

1 medium tomato, chopped

2-4 tablespoons snipped cilantro

8 whole wheat tortillas

shredded light cheddar cheese (optional)

salsa (optional)

> **Nutrition:**
>
> | 402 calories | 40 g protein |
> | 48 g carbs | 10 g fat |
> | 3 g sat. fat | 82 g cholesterol |
> | 502 mg sodium | 5 g fiber |

In a large skillet, add fat-free dressing and lime juice. Cook and stir onion strips for 1 minute. Add peppers; cook and stir until tender, about 1 more minute. Add meat. Cook and stir until meat is cooked through. Add chopped tomato and cilantro. Cook and stir until heated through. Serve with whole wheat tortillas. Garnish if desired with salsa and cheese.

Timesaving Tip: Purchase turkey or chicken bits: they will save you a lot of cutting-board time.

*To make this vegan, replace the meat with baked tofu strips and omit cheese.

Freezer Breakfast Bars (serves 8)

These are especially refreshing for a summer breakfast.

nonstick vegetable spray

2 1/2 cups Grape-Nuts or other
nugget-type cereal

3 tablespoon honey

2 8-oz. containers of nonfat berry
yogurt

1 cup berries (raspberries, strawberries, or boysenberries)

2/3 cup nonfat dry milk

> **Nutrition:**
>
> | 225 calories | 9 g protein |
> | 50 g carbs | 0 g fat |
> | 0 g sat. fat | 2 g cholesterol |
> | 304 mg sodium | 4 g fiber |

Lightly coat an 8" × 8" square pan with nonstick vegetable spray. Line pan with about 3/4 cup cereal. In a blender or food processor, combine honey, yogurt, fruit, and nonfat dry milk. Blend until smooth. Fold in 1 cup cereal. Pour yogurt mixture into pan. Top with remaining 3/4 cup cereal. Freeze for at least 4 hours or until firm. Cut into rectangles (they will look like ice-cream sandwiches).

Timesaving Tip: Keep these on hand, always ready when you are.

CHAPTER 13

Creating 60-Second Specials

"I don't have time for breakfast."—Corporate attorney

Can you squeeze just one minute into your busy schedule? All too often I hear the lament, "I don't have time to make breakfast . . . lunch . . . dinner." That's why I developed the 60-second meal. This chapter has 40 recipes that take one minute or less to make. The old "I don't have time" excuse is no longer valid.

The speediest one-minute meal is the Quickie, designed for breakneck nutrition when you're really pressed for time. The Quickie is simply a glass of nonfat milk followed by an orange juice chaser; it takes all of 19 seconds to prepare. You can do that! This combination may not seem like a meal, but it supplies about 30 percent of daily calcium needs and over 100 percent of the vitamin C requirements for women and 91 percent for men.

I have developed and tested these mini-meals to make sure that they can indeed be made in under 60 seconds and, of course, that they taste good, too! For additional nutritional value, you can combine these mini-meals with the grazing snacks in chapter 2.

Don't worry about measuring the ingredients. The eyeball technique ("it looks like a cup") will suffice. The measurements are just a guide, but they also serve as the basis for the nutritional information provided. Remember to have all ingredients assembled so you can speed through these recipes. The preparation time is based on ingredients purchased in the form they are called for. For example, buy your cheese already grated. You can certainly grate your own; it just requires a little more time. Each recipe makes one serving unless otherwise noted. An asterisk denotes vegan variations.

Tropical Wake-Up Smoothie

Prep time: 50 seconds

1/2 cup frozen fruit (banana, pine-
    apple, or mango chunks)
1 cup nonfat yogurt (tropical flavor)
1/4 cup orange juice

Nutrition:	
304 calories	13 g protein
64 g carbs	1 g fat
0 g sat. fat	4 g cholesterol
156 mg sodium	2 g fiber

   Mix all ingredients in a blender
until smooth.

*To make this vegan, use soy yogurt.

Hula Bagel

Prep time: 46 seconds

1 whole wheat bagel, sliced
1/3 cup low-fat ricotta cheese
1/4 cup crushed pineapple, drained
dash nutmeg

Nutrition:	
378 calories	21 g protein
65 g carbs	5 g fat
2 g sat. fat	24 g cholesterol
491 mg sodium	9 g fiber

   Combine ricotta cheese, crushed
pineapple, and nutmeg. Spread mixture on bagel halves.

Stuffed Cantaloupe

Prep time: 25 seconds

1/2 cantaloupe, seeds removed
1/2 cup nonfat cottage cheese
dash cinnamon

Nutrition:	
174 calories	17 g protein
26 g carbs	1 g fat
0 g sat. fat	10 g cholesterol
394 mg sodium	3 g fiber

   Scoop cottage cheese into hollow
section of melon. Sprinkle with cinnamon.

Bagel Melt

Prep time: 54 seconds

1 whole wheat bagel, sliced
2 slices low-fat cheese

Nutrition:	
350 calories	24 g protein
48 g carbs	7 g fat
4 g sat. fat	19 g cholesterol
745 mg sodium	8 g fiber

   Place cheese between bagel halves.
Microwave until cheese is melted.

Banana Roll-Up

Prep time: 60 seconds

2 teaspoons natural-style peanut
   butter
1/2 banana
1 teaspoon honey
1 tablespoon wheat germ
2 tablespoons nugget-type cereal
1/2 teaspoon pumpkin pie spice

Nutrition:	
215 calories	7 g protein
37 g carbs	7 g fat
1 g sat. fat	0 g cholesterol
97 mg sodium	4 g fiber

Spread peanut butter on banana until covered. Drizzle honey over the peanut butter-coated banana. Combine the wheat germ, cereal, and pumpkin pie spice on a paper plate or wax paper. Roll the banana in the wheat germ mixture until evenly coated.

Zippy Turkey Hoagie

Prep time: 35 seconds

1 deli-style whole wheat roll or hamburger bun
2 teaspoons fat-free Italian dressing
1-oz. slice turkey breast
1-oz. slice low-fat cheese
1 green lettuce leaf

Nutrition:	
319 calories	22 g protein
39 g carbs	8 g fat
3 g sat. fat	30 g cholesterol
641 mg sodium	5 g fiber

Spread dressing on roll. Layer turkey, cheese, and lettuce.

Submarine Cheese Melt

Prep time: 59 seconds

1 deli-style whole wheat roll or hamburger bun
2 teaspoons fat-free Italian dressing
1 oz. low-fat cheddar cheese
1 oz. low-fat Swiss cheese
3 tablespoons shredded lettuce
2 tomato slices

Nutrition:	
340 calories	24 g protein
42 g carbs	10 g fat
5 g sat. fat	30 g cholesterol
756 mg sodium	5 g fiber

Split roll into an open-faced butterfly. Spread dressing on each half. Add cheese to each half. Microwave until cheese starts to melt. Add the lettuce and tomato.

Lox and Bagel

Prep time: 47 seconds

1 whole wheat bagel, sliced
2 tablespoons light cream cheese
1 oz. lox or smoked salmon

Spread cream cheese on bagel. Top with lox or salmon.

Nutrition:	
323 calories	20 g protein
53 g carbs	5 g fat
2 g sat. fat	17 g cholesterol
787 mg sodium	9 g fiber

Pita Chili Melt

Prep time: 59 seconds

1/2 large (or whole small) whole
   wheat pita
1/2 cup canned pinto beans
2 tablespoons shredded low-fat
   cheddar cheese
1 tablespoon diced green chili

Put beans, cheese and chili into pita bread. Microwave until cheese melts.

*To make this vegan, omit the cheddar cheese.

Nutrition:	
315 calories	21 g protein
44 g carbs	7 g fat
4 g sat. fat	20 g cholesterol
719 mg sodium	11 g fiber

Hummus (Savory Chickpea Spread) and Pita

Prep time: 58 seconds

1 can (15 1/2 oz.) chickpeas
   (reserve 1/4 cup liquid)
2 tablespoons pesto sauce (ready-
   made in the deli section)
2 tablespoons tahini (sesame paste)
   or peanut butter
1 small whole wheat pita

In a blender or food processor, puree the chickpeas, reserved liquid, pesto, and tahini until smooth. While chickpeas are blending, cut pita into triangles. Serve hummus as a dip or spread.

Nutrition (1 serving = 1 pita and 1/4 cup hummus):	
303 calories	12 g protein
43 g carbs	10.5 g fat
2 g sat. fat	2 g cholesterol
630 mg sodium	8 g fiber

Tortilla Pinwheels

Prep time: 48 seconds

2 leaves green leaf lettuce
2 thin slices deli-cut turkey
1/2 tomato, sliced
1 whole wheat tortilla

Nutrition:	
180 calories	12 g protein
22 g carbs	5 g fat
2 g sat. fat	21 g cholesterol
206 mg sodium	4 g fiber

Layer lettuce, then turkey, and finally sliced tomato on tortilla. Roll up like a burrito. Insert 4 toothpicks to prevent unrolling. Then slice into 4 pinwheels (each with a toothpick). This simple but elegant recipe can also be used for quick appetizers.

Peanut Butter Banana Smoothie

Prep time: 57 seconds

1 cup nonfat milk
1 1/2 tablespoons natural-style chunky peanut butter
1 frozen banana (best frozen in thin slices for quick mixing)
1 teaspoon vanilla extract

Nutrition:	
340 calories	15 g protein
44 g carbs	13 g fat
2 g sat. fat	4 g cholesterol
129 mg sodium	4 g fiber

Mix all ingredients in a blender until smooth.

*To make this vegan, use vanilla soy milk and omit the vanilla extract.

Mini Gouda Artichoke Baguette

Prep time: 60 seconds

1 mini reduced-fat Gouda or Bonbel cheese
1 small (6-inch) baguette, split in half
2 marinated artichoke hearts, chopped

Nutrition:	
232 calories	13 g protein
34 g carbs	5 g fat
3 g sat. fat	15 g cholesterol
718 mg sodium	2 g fiber

Slice cheese thinly and place on each half of bread. Top with chopped artichoke hearts. Microwave until cheese is slightly melted.

Greek Stuffed Pita

Prep time: 60 seconds

2 tablespoons chopped raw spinach
2 tablespoons crumbled feta cheese
1 tablespoon fat-free cream cheese
1/2 large (or whole small) whole wheat pita

Nutrition:	
311 calories	18 g protein
52 g carbs	5 g fat
3 g sat. fat	18 g cholesterol
639 mg sodium	7 g fiber

In a small bowl, combine spinach and cheeses. Stuff into pita. Microwave until cheese is melted.

Mexican Pita Pizza

Prep time: 60 seconds

1 small whole wheat pita
1 tablespoon salsa
1/4 cup fat-free refried beans
1 oz. low-fat pepper jack or jack cheese

Nutrition:	
228 calories	14 g protein
31 g carbs	6 g fat
4 g sat. fat	20 g cholesterol
764 mg sodium	6 g fiber

Spread salsa evenly over top of pita. Add beans and top with cheese. Microwave until cheese is melted.

Peach Smoothie

Prep time: 53 seconds

1 cup frozen, unsweetened peaches
1/2 cup nonfat vanilla or peach yogurt
1/4 cup nonfat milk
1 teaspoon vanilla extract
dash nutmeg

Nutrition:	
210 calories	9 g protein
44 g carbs	0 g fat
0 g sat. fat	4 g cholesterol
102 mg sodium	3 g fiber

Combine all ingredients in blender until smooth.

*To make this vegan, use soy yogurt and soy milk.

The Quickie

Prep time: 19 seconds

1 cup nonfat milk
1 cup orange juice

Pour milk into cup and drink. Pour juice into glass and drink. Off you go!

*To make this vegan, use soy milk.

Nutrition:

198 calories	10 g protein
38 g carbs	1 g fat
0 g sat. fat	4 g cholesterol
128 mg sodium	0 g fiber

English Muffin Melt

Prep time: 60 seconds

1 whole wheat English muffin, split
1-oz. slice low-fat Swiss cheese

Place 1/2 slice of cheese on each muffin half. Bake in broiler or microwave until cheese melts. For variety, top with one slice of Canadian bacon.

Nutrition:

255 calories	17 g protein
41 g carbs	4 g fat
1 g sat. fat	10 g cholesterol
712 mg sodium	10 g fiber

Curried Chicken Sandwich

Prep time: 58 seconds

1/4 cup leftover chopped chicken
   or 1/2 (5-oz.) can of white chunk
   chicken
1/4 teaspoon curry powder
1/2 teaspoon dried mustard
   powder
1 stalk celery, chopped
1 tablespoon light mayonnaise
2 slices whole wheat bread

Nutrition:

300 calories	19 g protein
36 g carbs	10 g fat
2 g sat. fat	30 g cholesterol
529 mg sodium	5 g fiber

Combine chicken, spices, celery, and mayonnaise and mix well. Spread on bread.

Pita Surprise

Prep time: 28 seconds

1/2 large whole wheat pita
1/2 cup leftovers

   Put leftovers in pita.

> **Nutrition:**
> too variable to analyze

Ak-Mak and Cheese

Prep time: 11 seconds

1 oz. low-fat cheese
4 Ak-Mak or other whole-grain
   crackers

   Simply place a bite of cheese on each cracker. My favorite cheese to use is low-fat smoked Gouda.

*To make this vegan, use soy cheese.

> **Nutrition:**
> 146 calories   11 g protein
> 11 g carbs   7 g fat
> 1 g sat. fat   20 g cholesterol
> 712 mg sodium   2 g fiber

Turkey Roll-Up

Prep time: 20 seconds

2 slices turkey ham
1 leaf romaine lettuce
1 carrot stick

   Place turkey evenly over lettuce leaf. Add carrot. Roll up like a burrito.

> **Nutrition:**
> 105 calories   12 g protein
> 8 g carbs   3 g fat
> 1 g sat. fat   32 g cholesterol
> 591 mg sodium   2 g fiber

Spiced Peanut Butter and Apple Wedges

Prep time: 30 seconds

1 tablespoon natural-style peanut
   butter
1 tablespoon fat-free ricotta
1/4 teaspoon cinnamon
1 medium apple, cut into wedges

   In a small bowl or cup, mix together the peanut butter, ricotta, and cinnamon.

> **Nutrition:**
> 186 calories   6 g protein
> 26 g carbs   8 g fat
> 1 g sat. fat   2 g cholesterol
> 9 mg sodium   4 g fiber

Timesaving Tip: The fastest way to cut apples is with an apple slicer, which automatically cores and cuts the apple into even wedges.

Orange Reveille

Prep time: 59 seconds

6-oz. can orange juice concentrate, thawed

2 cans (12 oz.) water

1/4 cup nonfat dried milk powder

9 ice cubes

1 teaspoon vanilla extract

Nutrition (1 serving):

341 calories	10 g protein
74 g carbs	0 g fat
0 g sat. fat	3 g cholesterol
98 mg sodium	1 g fiber

Mix all ingredients in a blender until smooth. Makes 2 servings.

Tortilla Sandwich

Prep time: 48 seconds

2 whole wheat tortillas

1/4 cup chicken (or leftover protein source)

1 tablespoon low-fat cheese

2 lettuce leaves

Nutrition:

326 calories	22 g protein
37 g carbs	10 g fat
4 g sat. fat	40 g cholesterol
502 mg sodium	6 g fiber

Place chicken, cheese, and lettuce on one tortilla. Cover with the remaining tortilla. Microwave just until the cheese melts. Cut into triangles.

Basic Sandwich

Prep time: 42 seconds

2 slices whole wheat bread

2 slices or 1/4 cup tuna, chicken, turkey, or other protein source

2 slices tomato

1 romaine lettuce leaf

Nutrition:

292 calories	24 g protein
34 g carbs	7 g fat
2 g sat. fat	41 g cholesterol
405 mg sodium	5 g fiber

Place ingredients between bread.

Pita Salad

Prep time: 60 seconds

1/2 cup salad
1 oz. firm tofu, cut into cubes
1 tablespoon light salad dressing
1/2 large (or whole small) whole
   wheat pita

> **Nutrition:**
>
> | | |
> |---|---|
> | 189 calories | 10 g protein |
> | 29 g carbs | 5 g fat |
> | 1 g sat. fat | 0 g cholesterol |
> | 368 mg sodium | 4 g fiber |

Toss together the tofu, salad, and dressing. Stuff mixture into pita.

Quesadilla

Prep time: 58 seconds

2 tablespoons shredded low-fat
   cheddar cheese
1 tablespoon salsa
1 teaspoon cilantro
1 whole wheat tortilla

> **Nutrition:**
>
> | | |
> |---|---|
> | 196 calories | 12 g protein |
> | 19 g carbs | 8 g fat |
> | 4 g sat. fat | 20 g cholesterol |
> | 563 mg sodium | 3 g fiber |

Place cheese, salsa, and cilantro on tortilla. Microwave until cheese melts.

*To make this vegan, use soy cheese. Vegans should check the whole wheat tortilla for the source of fat.

Cereal and Milk

Prep time: 31 seconds

1 oz. (1/2 to 1 cup) whole-grain
   cereal
3/4 cup nonfat milk
5 strawberries or 1/2 banana,
   sliced

> **Nutrition:**
>
> | | |
> |---|---|
> | 205 calories | 10 g protein |
> | 44 g carbs | 1 g fat |
> | 0 g sat. fat | 3 g cholesterol |
> | 252 mg sodium | 4 g fiber |

Place cereal, milk, and fruit in bowl.

Nutrition varies with cereal used.

*To make this vegan, use soy milk.

Turkey Bagel

Prep time: 41 seconds

2 oz. sliced turkey breast
1 romaine lettuce leaf
1 whole wheat bagel, sliced

Put turkey and lettuce and bagel.

Nutrition (1 serving):
362 calories   28.5 g protein
52 g carbs   6 g fat
2 g sat. fat   41 g cholesterol
494 mg sodium   9 g fiber

Banana Health Shake

Prep time: 60 seconds

1 frozen banana (best frozen in thin slices for quick mixing)
1/4 cup nonfat dried powdered milk
1/2 cup orange juice
1 teaspoon vanilla extract
dash nutmeg
5 ice cubes

Mix all ingredients in a blender until smooth.

Nutrition:
231 calories   8 g protein
49 g carbs   1 g fat
0 g sat. fat   3 g cholesterol
96 mg sodium   3 g fiber

Rice Cake Crunch

Prep time: 49 seconds

1 teaspoon fat-free cream cheese
1 large rice cake
2 oz. sliced chicken breast
5 cucumber slices
dash paprika

Spread cream cheese on rice cake. Top with chicken, cucumber, and paprika.

Nutrition:
136 calories   19 g protein
8 g carbs   2 g fat
1 g sat. fat   49 g cholesterol
92 mg sodium   0 g fiber

Strawberry Yogurt Frappe

Prep time: 57 seconds

7 frozen strawberries
1/4 cup milk
1 cup nonfat strawberry yogurt
dash vanilla extract

Nutrition:	
183 calories	13 g protein
33 g carbs	1 g fat
0 g sat. fat	8 g cholesterol
147 mg sodium	3 g fiber

Mix all ingredients in a blender until smooth.

*To make this vegan, use soy yogurt.

Quick Pizza

Prep time: 59 seconds

1 whole wheat English muffin, split
2 tablespoons spaghetti sauce
2 tablespoons shredded low-fat
    mozzarella cheese

Nutrition:	
234 calories	13 g protein
31 g carbs	6 g fat
3 g sat. fat	16 g cholesterol
485 mg sodium	3 g fiber

Spread spaghetti sauce on both slices of English muffin. Top with cheese. Microwave until cheese is melted.

Pita Pan

Prep time: 24 seconds

1/2 large (or whole small) whole
    wheat pita
1 tablespoon peanut butter
1/2 banana, sliced

Nutrition:	
266 calories	9 g protein
42 g carbs	9 g fat
1 g sat. fat	0 g cholesterol
241 mg sodium	5 g fiber

Spread peanut butter inside pita. Add banana slices.

Fiesta Bean Burrito

Prep time: 59 seconds

1/2 cup fat-free refried beans
1 whole wheat tortilla
1 tablespoon salsa
1 teaspoon chopped cilantro
    (optional)

Nutrition (1 serving):	
160 calories	6 g protein
28 g carbs	3 g fat
1 g sat. fat	0 g cholesterol
625 mg sodium	7 g fiber

Spread beans over tortilla. Add salsa and cilantro, if desired. Microwave until warm, about 40 seconds. Roll tortilla and mixture into a burrito.

*Vegans should check the whole wheat tortilla for the source of fat.

Peanut Butter Melt

Prep time: 58 seconds

1 slice whole wheat bread
1/2 banana
2 teaspoons peanut butter

Nutrition:	
195 calories	6 g protein
31 g carbs	7 g fat
1 g sat. fat	0 g cholesterol
183 mg sodium	5 g fiber

Toast bread. While bread is toasting, slice banana. Spread peanut butter on toast and top with banana.

Peanut Butter Wrap

Prep time: 60 seconds

1 whole wheat tortilla
1 tablespoon peanut butter
1 tablespoon applesauce
1 tablespoon raisins
dash of cinnamon

Nutrition:	
241 calories	7 g protein
31 g carbs	11 g fat
2 g sat. fat	0 g cholesterol
183 mg sodium	5 g fiber

Warm tortilla in microwave (about 15 seconds). Spread peanut butter evenly on tortilla. Add applesauce and raisins. Roll up.

*Vegans should check the whole wheat tortilla for the source of fat.

Cottage Raisin Toast

Prep time: 60 seconds

1 slice raisin bread
1/4 cup nonfat cottage cheese
1 teaspoon raisins
dash cinnamon

> **Nutrition:**
> 113 calories   9 g protein
> 17 g carbs   1 g fat
> 0 g sat. fat   5 g cholesterol
> 274 mg sodium   1 g fiber

Toast bread. Spread cottage cheese on toast. Sprinkle with raisins and cinnamon.

Tuna Salad Pita

Prep time: 60 seconds

1/2 large (or whole small) whole
    wheat pita
1/4 cup shredded lettuce
1 mini (3-oz.) can of water-packed
    tuna
1 tablespoon light mayonnaise
dash pepper

> **Nutrition:**
> 280 calories   927 g protein
> 26 g carbs   8 g fat
> 1 g sat. fat   36 g cholesterol
> 673 mg sodium   3 g fiber

Line pita bread with lettuce. Combine tuna, mayonnaise, and pepper. Stuff tuna mixture into pita.

Surviving the Holidays

"I don't have enough time to wrap presents, let alone eat healthy during the holidays."—Stockbroker

Every year without fail, I get calls from reporters asking about how to survive the holidays. It's a tough season for most people to eat healthfully, between the time spent shopping and running to parties and the endless gifts of food and those once-a-year holiday treats. I love the holiday season and value my health, and the two don't need to be mutually exclusive. In this chapter I give strategies to make your holidays healthy without hassle. But first, see how you normally fare during the holidays by taking this quick quiz.

Holiday Quiz

1. Do you often feel obligated to have second helpings at holiday meals?

2. Do you nervously slurp down beverages at holiday gatherings when you're at a loss for something to say?

3. Do you sample cookie dough during holiday baking?

4. Do you feel obligated to eat every food gift you receive?

5. Do you take a food celibacy vow, only to devour mounds of holiday goodies?

6. Is the only exercise you get those mad dashes between stores and holiday meals?

7. At parties do you fill up on appetizers, but go ahead and eat a big meal even though you are full?

8. Do you plan to feast on anything you want because you plan to start dieting on January 1?

9. Do you skip meals before holiday parties to save time and calories?

10. Do you cope with the holidays by eating more food?

If you answered yes to two or more of these questions, this chapter is for you!

HOLIDAY WEIGHT GAIN

Don't assume that weight gain is a given during the holidays. For many years it was commonly accepted that people gain about five or more pounds during the holidays. But a study reported in the *New England Journal of Medicine* showed otherwise To evaluate holiday weight gain, researchers from the National Institutes of Health weighed 195 people during three time periods: preholiday, holiday season (mid-November to early January), and after the holiday period. They found that the average weight gain was about one pound. The philosophy of feasting during the holidays because tomorrow you diet, however, can truly make matters worse. The strategies in this chapter combined with regular exercise during the holidays will keep you healthy. But don't forget to keep the pleasure in the holiday season.

RICH HOLIDAY MEALS

There's no doubt that holiday meals are all dressed up, usually richer and with more fat. These strategies can help you avoid overindulging.

- Don't arrive to dinner on a ravenous stomach, as this can easily lead to overeating.
- There's no food you love that you can't have—any time of the year. This attitude makes holiday food less magnetic.
- Rather than scooping out a serving from each dish, choose the holiday foods you simply can't do without.
- Pass up food that you won't miss. For example, a roll with butter at mealtime is not likely to be missed, and forgoing it is not likely to lead to feelings of deprivation.
- Beware of lingering. When you are finished eating, remove your plate, put a napkin on your plate, or put your silverware on your plate to prevent unintentional nibbling at the table.
- If you eat more than you intended, let it go, rather than thinking you blew it. All-or-none thinking can lead to even more eating.

HOLIDAY FARE

Holidays are a time for celebrating, and more often than not, celebrating means food, a continuous smorgasbord of goodies! Sumptuous desserts, delicate little chocolates, roasted ham basted in brown sugar, eggnog and other holiday cocktails. And you have to be polite, right? The first sight of a candy cane or chocolate bunny makes many people dread inevitable holiday munching. But rest easy, there are ways to survive the feasts without foundering.

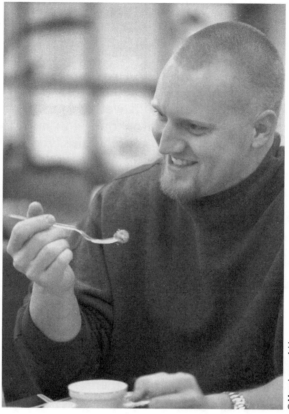

© Mary Langenfeld

It's okay to treat yourself on holidays! Just remember a little bite can go a long way.

Making the Rounds at Holiday Buffets

Buffets can be challenging anytime, but during the holidays the challenge can be doubled by the variety of food and the social factor. Several studies indicate that when we're exposed to a wider variety of foods at one sitting, we have a tendency to eat more. We are also likely to eat more when there are other people around: the more people present, the more we tend to eat. Here's what you can do to counter the holiday overeating effect:

- Carry on your conversations away from the buffet table; otherwise, it's all too easy to turn to food when searching for words.
- Focus on socializing at parties: introduce yourself to others rather than making food the primary focus.
- Offer to bring a dish, and make it a healthy one.
- Plan to make one trip to the buffet table, unless you are still hungry.

Holiday Cocktail Parties

Cocktail parties are also culprits. The following tips should help you be sociable and sated.

- Try not to arrive on an empty stomach, as an empty stomach absorbs alcohol more quickly. Alcohol is the only digestible substance that gets absorbed in the stomach rather than in the intestine.
- Be careful of unconscious nibbling on appetizers or holiday goodies that you don't truly want.
- Try making one drink last the whole party, or try spacing alcoholic drinks with noncaloric beverages such as mineral water.

Holiday Food Gifts

Holidays are the time for giving. As we ponder what to get whom and how much to spend, very often we turn to food, which is easy, convenient, and something everyone likes. Whether you are giving or receiving, food is an alluring way to say thanks. Graciously accepting a food gift doesn't mean you have to eat it (unless you want to). Eat some, if you wish, freeze the rest, or share your bounty at the office or with neighbors. What do you do with a food basket with cheeses and canned meats that you really don't want? Try donating the gifts to a local food bank.

HOLIDAY HOSTING

You're throwing a party, and everything has to be just right, especially the food. It's enough to keep track of your own nibbling, much less providing healthy snacks for everyone else. But if you plan ahead, making sure that there are plenty of options for those who want to eat healthfully, it's really quite simple!

I once hosted a holiday party that had a cascade of assorted fruits that occupied the whole table (it was catered and quite a lovely arrangement). It was the most talked about and enjoyed food option! Here are some ideas for healthy timesavers that can be purchased at your local grocery store:

- Chicken satays
- Veggie platter
- Fruit platter
- Hummus dip with pita wedges
- Cranberry relish
- Roasted turkey
- Lean deli meat platter: roast beef, turkey slices, chicken slices

And what if you're a guest, especially a relative? Visiting any relative can add special challenges to healthy eating: family pressure can be worse than peer pressure. For the adoring relative who loves to pamper you with home-baked treats, practice polite responses when you don't feel like eating, such as, "I'm so full I couldn't possibly eat another bite. Could I take it home?"

HOLIDAY BAKING

One of our family traditions is to bake holiday treats, but I usually try to add some healthy twist, such as substituting applesauce for oil in ginger-bread, using light butter instead of regular butter, scattering nuts on top of baked goods rather than mixing them in, and omitting the sugar from spiced apple cider that is heavy on the spices.

Visions of Sugarplums Dance in Their Heads

Visions of sugarplums and grandma's fudge make you drool, and for good reason—they are absolutely delicious. So make the most of those holidays treats.

- Be sure to truly savor each and every bite of a holiday treat.
- Remember that there is nothing special about ordinary candies dressed up in holiday colors.
- If you don't love it, don't eat it.
- Special tip for boxes of chocolate: If you select a piece that you don't like, politely toss it rather than eat it!

No matter where you are, or how tight your schedule is, you are only one bite away from healthy eating. Remember: progress, not perfection, is what truly matters. One snack, one meal, or one day of eating will not make or break your health. It's the consistent pattern that counts.

Regardless of your lifestyle or eating habits (be it fast food, frozen food, or restaurant food), it is possible to eat nutritionally in a minimal amount of time. You *can* eat on the run and eat healthy.

APPENDIX A:
Fast-Food Nutritional Charts

Item	Calories	Fat (g)	Sat. fat (g)	Cholesterol (mg)	Protein (g)	Carbs (g)	Sodium (mg)
Arby's							
Roast beef sandwiches							
Arby's Melt w/Cheddar	340	15	5	70	16	36	890
Arby-Q	360	14	4	70	16	40	1,530
Beef 'N Cheddar	480	24	8	90	23	43	1,240
Big Montana	630	32	15	155	47	41	2,080
Giant Roast Beef	480	23	10	110	32	41	1,440
Junior Roast Beef	310	13	4.5	70	16	34	740
Regular Roast Beef	350	16	6	85	21	34	950
Super Roast Beef	470	23	7	85	22	47	1,130
Other sandwiches							
Chicken Bacon 'N Swiss	610	33	8	110	31	49	1,550
Chicken Breast Fillet	540	30	5	90	24	47	1,160
Chicken Cordon Bleu	620	35	8	120	34	47	1,820
Grilled Chicken Deluxe	440	22	4	110	29	37	1,050
Roast Chicken Club	520	28	7	115	29	38	1,440
Hot Ham 'N Cheese	340	13	4.5	90	23	35	1,450
Sub sandwiches							
French Dip	440	18	8	100	28	42	1,680
Hot Ham 'N Swiss	530	27	8	110	29	45	1,860
Italian	780	53	15	120	29	49	2,450
Philly Beef 'N Swiss	700	42	15	130	36	46	1,940
Roast Beef	760	48	16	130	35	47	2,230
Turkey	630	37	9	100	26	51	2,170
Arby's Market Fresh sandwiches							
Roast Beef & Swiss	810	42	13	130	37	73	1,780
Roast Ham & Swiss	730	34	8	125	36	74	2,180
Roast Chicken Caesar	820	38	9	140	43	75	2,160
Roast Turkey & Swiss	760	33	6	130	43	75	1,920
Arby's Market Fresh salads (dressings not included)							
Turkey Club Salad	350	21	10	90	33	9	920
Caesar Salad	90	4	2.5	10	7	8	170
Grilled Chicken Caesar	230	8	3.5	80	33	8	920
Chicken Finger Salad	570	34	9	65	30	39	1,300
Caesar Side Salad	45	2	1	5	4	4	85

Item	Calories	Fat (g)	Sat. fat (g)	Cholesterol (mg)	Protein (g)	Carbs (g)	Sodium (mg)
Light menu							
Light Grilled Chicken	280	5	1.5	55	29	30	1,170
Light Roast Chicken Deluxe	260	5	1	40	23	33	1,010
Light Roast Turkey Deluxe	260	5	0.5	40	23	33	980
Salads							
Garden Salad	70	1	0	0	4	14	45
Grilled Chicken Salad	210	4.5	1.5	65	30	14	800
Roast Chicken Salad	160	2.5	0	40	20	15	700
Side Salad	25	0	0	0	2	5	20
Sides							
Curly Fries, SM	310	15	3.5	0	4	39	770
Curly Fries, M	400	20	5	0	5	50	990
Curly Fries, LG	620	30	7	0	8	78	1,540
Cheddar Curly Fries	460	24	6	5	6	54	1,290
Homestyle Fries, child size	220	10	2.5	0	3	32	430
Homestyle Fries, SM	300	13	3.5	0	3	42	570
Homestyle Fries, M	370	16	4	0	4	53	710
Homestyle Fries, LG	560	24	6	0	6	79	1,070
Potato Cakes (2)	250	16	4	0	2	26	490
Chicken Finger 4-Pack	640	38	8	70	31	42	1,590
Chicken Finger Snack	580	32	7	35	19	55	1,450
Jalapeno Bites	330	21	9	40	7	30	670
Mozzarella Sticks	470	29	14	60	18	34	1,330
Onion Petals	410	24	3.5	0	4	43	300
Baked Potato, with butter and sour cream	500	24	15	55	8	65	170
Broccoli 'N Cheddar Baked Potato	540	24	12	50	12	71	680
Deluxe Baked Potato	650	34	20	90	20	67	750
Desserts							
Apple turnover	420	16	4.5	0	4	65	230
Cherry turnover	410	16	4.5	0	4	63	250
Breakfast items							
Biscuit w/Butter	280	17	4	0	5	27	780
Biscuit w/Ham	330	20	5	30	12	28	830
Biscuit w/Sausage	460	33	9	25	12	28	300
Biscuit w/Bacon	360	24	7	10	9	27	220
Croissant w/Ham	310	19	11	50	13	29	1,130
Croissant w/Sausage	440	32	15	45	13	29	600
Croissant w/Bacon	340	23	13	30	10	28	520
Sourdough w/Ham	390	6	1	30	19	67	1,570

Item	Calories	Fat (g)	Sat. fat (g)	Cholesterol (mg)	Protein (g)	Carbs (g)	Sodium (mg)
Sourdough w/Sausage	520	19	5	25	19	67	1,040
Sourdough w/Bacon	420	10	2.5	10	16	66	960
Add egg	110	9	2	175	5	2	170
Add slice of Swiss cheese	45	3	2	10	3	0	220
French Toastix (no syrup)	370	17	4	0	7	48	440
Condiments							
Arby's Sauce	15	0	0	0	0	4	180
Au Jus Sauce	5	0.05	0.02	0	0.3	0.89	386
BBQ Dipping Sauce	40	0	0	0	0	10	350
BBQ Vinaigrette Dressing	140	11	1.5	0	0	9	660
Blue Cheese Dressing	300	31	6	45	2	3	580
Bronco Berry Sauce	90	0	0	0	0	23	35
Buttermilk Ranch Dressing	360	39	6	5	1	2	490
Buttermilk Ranch Dressing, reduced calorie	60	0	0	0	1	13	750
Caesar Dressing	310	34	5	60	1	1	470
Croutons, Cheese and Garlic	100	6.25	N/A	N/A	2.5	10	138
Croutons, Seasoned	30	15	0	0	1	5	70
French Toast Syrup	130	0	0	0	0	32	45
German Mustard	5	0	0	0	0	0	60
Honey French Dressing	290	24	4	0	0	18	410
Honey Mustard Dipping Sauce	130	12	1.5	10	0	5	160
Horsey Sauce	60	5	0.5	5	0	3	150
Italian Dressing, reduced calorie	25	1	1	0	0	3	1,030
Italian Parmesan Dressing	240	24	4	0	1	4	950
Ketchup	10	0	0	0	0	2	100
Marinara Sauce	35	1	0	0	1	4	260
Mayonnaise	90	10	1.5	10	0	0	65
Mayonnaise, light, cholesterol free	20	1.5	0	0	0	1	110
Tangy Southwest Sauce	250	26	4.5	30	0	3	290
Thousand Island Dressing	290	28	4.5	35	1	9	480
Beverages							
Milk (2%)	120	5	3	20	8	12	120
Orange juice	140	0	0	0	1	34	0
Hot chocolate	110	1	0.5	0	2	23	120
Chocolate shake	480	16	8	45	10	84	370
Jamocha shake	470	15	7	45	10	82	390
Strawberry shake	500	13	8	15	11	87	340
Vanilla shake	470	15	7	45	10	83	360

Item	Calories	Fat (g)	Sat. fat (g)	Cholesterol (mg)	Protein (g)	Carbs (g)	Sodium (mg)
Baja Fresh							
Baja Fresh Burritos							
Baja Steak	847	41	N/A	140	59	60	N/A
Baja Chicken	809	36	N/A	145	57	59	N/A
Mexicano Steak	933	25	N/A	90	57	120	N/A
Mexicano Chicken	895	20	N/A	95	55	120	N/A
Bean & Cheese	867	31	N/A	68	43	102	N/A
Bean, Cheese, & Steak	1,090	40	N/A	158	78	102	N/A
Bean, Cheese, & Chicken	1,052	35	N/A	163	76	102	N/A
Burrito Ultimo Steak	1,109	50	N/A	170	63	90	N/A
Burrito Ultimo Chicken	1,070	45	N/A	175	57	90	N/A
Grilled Vegetarian	834	37	N/A	80	32	84	N/A
Burrito Dos Manos Steak	1,646	65	N/A	183	80	173	N/A
Burrito Dos Manos Chicken	1,608	60	N/A	188	78	173	N/A
Baja Style Tacos							
Baja Steak	106	3	N/A	25	11	20	N/A
Baja Chicken	90	2	N/A	23	10	20	N/A
Baja Shrimp	90	3	N/A	55	9	20	N/A
Baja Mahi Mahi Taco	216	11	N/A	41	13	24	N/A
Baja Fish Taco	143	9	N/A	22	7	21	N/A
Taco Chilito							
Steak	373	15	N/A	56	21	35	N/A
Chicken	363	13	N/A	57	21	35	N/A
Taquitos							
Steak	483	45	N/A	37	21	65	N/A
Chicken	514	45	N/A	41	22	65	N/A
Baja Fajita Combo (includes beans, sour cream, and guacamole; does not include tortilla)							
Steak	842	36	N/A	104	60	101	N/A
Chicken	777	31	N/A	94	55	101	N/A
Quesadilla							
Cheese Quesadilla	1,011	62	N/A	151	46	59	N/A
Steak	1,211	70	N/A	234	76	60	N/A
Chicken	1,172	66	N/A	235	78	59	N/A
Mini Cheese Quesadita	636	22	N/A	38	30	94	N/A
Mini Steak Quesadita	692	25	N/A	61	38	94	N/A
Mini Chicken Quesadita	682	23	N/A	62	39	94	N/A
Nachos							
Cheese Nachos	1,735	98	N/A	161	51	154	N/A
Steak Nachos	1,958	107	N/A	251	84	154	N/A
Chicken Nachos	1,920	102	N/A	256	86	154	N/A
Torta							
Steak	903	48	N/A	119	49	72	N/A
Chicken	865	43	N/A	124	47	72	N/A

Item	Calories	Fat (g)	Sat. fat (g)	Cholesterol (mg)	Protein (g)	Carbs (g)	Sodium (mg)
Baja Ensalada							
Steak	905	63	N/A	118	48	37	N/A
Chicken	857	57	N/A	124	51	38	N/A
Tostada							
Steak	847	41	N/A	140	59	60	N/A
Chicken	809	36	N/A	145	57	59	N/A
Mini Tostadita	785	29	N/A	78	45	91	N/A
Blimpie							
Cold subs							
6" Best Sub on White	410	13	5	50	39	47	1,480
6" Best Sub on Wheat	410	13	5	50	39	47	1,480
6" Cheese Trio Sub on White	490	23	12	55	25	48	1,130
6" Cheese Trio Sub on Wheat	490	23	12	55	26	48	1,110
6" Club Sub on White	370	10	4.5	30	23	48	1,200
6" Club Sub on Wheat	370	11	4.5	30	23	48	1,180
6" Ham, Salami, & Provolone Sub on White	480	20	8	55	24	49	1,370
6" Ham, Salami, & Provolone Sub on Wheat	450	20	8	55	24	47	1,350
6" Ham & Swiss Sub on White	410	14	7	50	25	48	1,050
6" Ham & Swiss Sub on Wheat	400	14	7	50	26	46	1,040
6" Tuna Sub on White	660	44	8	55	18	51	880
6" Tuna Sub on Wheat	650	45	6	55	18	49	860
6" Turkey Sub on White	330	6	1.5	0	19	48	1,200
6" Turkey Sub on Wheat	330	7	1.5	0	19	48	1,190
6" Roast Beef Sub on White	390	7	3	65	37	47	1,370
6" Roast Beef Sub on Wheat	390	8	3	65	37	45	1,380
Hot subs							
Steak & Cheese	550	26	3.5	70	27	51	1,080
Grilled Chicken	400	9	2	30	28	52	950
Italian Meatball	500	22	8	25	23	52	970
Smokey Cheddar Beef Melt	380	12	6	50	23	42	1,200
Roast Turkey Cordon Bleu	430	14	6	60	29	43	1,180
ChikMax on White	483	12	1	0	33.6	69.9	1,293
ChikMax on Wheat	495	13	1	0	25.8	69.3	1,370
Grille Max on White	413	6	1	5	18.1	71.9	823.2
Grille Max on Wheat	425	7	1	5	18.8	71.3	900.4
VegiMax on White	403	7	0.5	0	24	61	980
VegiMax on Wheat	415	8	0.5	0	24	60	1,050

Item	Calories	Fat (g)	Sat. fat (g)	Cholesterol (mg)	Protein (g)	Carbs (g)	Sodium (mg)
Hot subs (continued)							
MexiMax on White	393	5	1	0	25	66	1,003
MexiMax on Wheat	405	6	1	0	25	65	1,080
Wraps							
Chicken Caesar Wrap	610	31	6	35	26	56	1,770
Southwestern Wrap	590	28	7	75	28	56	1,990
Zesty Italian Wrap	530	22	7	45	24	59	1,850
Sides							
Antipasto Salad	200	11	5	50	19	9	950
Chef Salad	150	6	3	40	17	8	600
Club Salad	130	6	3	30	14	7	450
Ham & Swiss Cheese Salad	170	8	6	40	16	7	500
Italian Pasta Supreme Salad	180	7	1	0	3	20	840
Roast Beef Salad	120	2.5	1.5	25	19	8	480
Tossed Green Salad	35	0.5	0	0	2	7	20
Tuna Salad	130	1.5	0	45	22	7	400
Turkey Salad	90	0.5	0	25	15	8	580
Coleslaw (1/2 cup)	180	13	2	< 5	1	13	230
Macaroni Salad (2/3 cup)	360	25	4	10	4	25	660
Mustard Potato Salad (2/3 cup)	160	5	1	5	2	21	660
Potato Salad (2/3 cup)	270	19	3	10	2	19	560
Classic Chili with Beans & Beef (1 cup)	240	8	3.5	40	14	27	1,060
Chicken Noodle Soup (1 cup)	140	3	1	30	8	20	1,190
Chicken Soup with White & Wild Rice (1 cup)	230	12	2	30	10	21	1,210
Cream of Potato Soup (1 cup)	190	9	2.5	< 5	5	24	860
Classic Chili with Beans & Beef (1 cup)	240	8	3.5	40	14	27	1,060
Chicken Noodle Soup (1 cup)	140	3	1	30	8	20	1,190
Classic Chili with Beans & Beef (1 cup)	240	8	3.5	40	14	27	1,060
Chicken Noodle Soup (1 cup)	140	3	1	30	8	20	1,190
Chicken Soup with White & Wild Rice (1 cup)	230	12	2	30	10	21	1,210
Cream of Potato Soup (1 cup)	190	9	2.5	< 5	5	24	860

Item	Calories	Fat (g)	Sat. fat (g)	Cholesterol (mg)	Protein (g)	Carbs (g)	Sodium (mg)
Breads							
White Sub Roll (about 6")	240	3.5	1	0	8.5	43	490
Wheat Sub Roll (about 6")	235	4	1	0	9	40.5	475
Mission Traditional Wrap	301	7.5	1.6	0	7.8	47.9	761
Mission Spinach Herb Wrap	308	8	1.6	0	7.8	49	781
Mediterranean Flatbread	270	9	1.5	0	10	37	N/A
Veggie Sub Roll (about 6")	238.8	3.5	0.8	0	8.4	43.5	502.6
Marbled Rye Sub Roll (about 6")	246.4	2.5	0.6	0	9.5	47.3	586
Dressings and sauces							
Fat-Free Italian Dressing (1 fl. oz.)	20	0	0	0	0	5	670
Light Italian Dressing (1.5 fl. oz.)	20	1	0	0	0	3	810
Light Buttermilk Ranch Dressing (1.5 fl. oz.)	90	5	1	0	1	10	350
Blue Cheese Dressing (1 fl. oz.)	220	24	4	40	2	2	440
Buttermilk Ranch Dressing (1 fl. oz.)	270	29	4	5	0	1	360
Honey French Dressing (1 fl. oz.)	240	20	3	0	0	16	350
Thousand Island Dressing (1 fl. oz.)	210	21	3	25	0	7	360
Blimpie Special Sub Dressing (3/4 fl. oz.)	70	7	1	0	0	0	0
Blimpie Dressing (1 fl. oz.)	120	8	1	0	1	16	570
Guacamole (1 oz.)	194	17.5	2.7	< 1	1.8	7.4	468.1
Mayonnaise (1 tbsp.)	100	11	1.5	10	0	1	60
Toppings (per oz.)							
Lettuce	3.7	0	N/A	N/A	0.3	0.06	2.6
Tomato	6.3	0.5	N/A	N/A	0.3	1.3	1
Onions	10.9	0.5	N/A	N/A	0.4	2.5	2.8
Sweet peppers	10	0	N/A	N/A	0	5	75
Hot peppers	0	0	N/A	N/A	0	1	240
Jalapeno peppers	0	0	N/A	N/A	0	1	210
Red cabbage	8.9	0.5	N/A	N/A	0.6	2	0.2
Carrots	12	0.06	N/A	N/A	0.3	2.6	13.4
Baked goods							
Chocolate Chunk Cookie	201	10	6	15	2	26	201
Macadamia White Chunk Cookie	210	10	5	20	2	26	140

Item	Calories	Fat (g)	Sat. fat (g)	Cholesterol (mg)	Protein (g)	Carbs (g)	Sodium (mg)
Baked goods (continued)							
Oatmeal Raisin Cookie	191	8	2	15	3	27	201
Peanut Butter Cookie	221	12	5	15	4	27	201
Sugar Cookie	330	17	4.5	30	3	24.2	290
Fudge Brownies	243.2	10.8	N/A	20	2.6	33.6	168.8
Banana Nut Muffin	472	23	N/A	55	8	55	442
Blueberry Muffin	412	18	N/A	55	7	55	452
Bran & Raisin Muffin	442	18	N/A	20	7	64	502
Cinnamon Roll	631	25	N/A	0	9	90	692
White Roll Icing (1 oz.)	97	0.56	N/A	0	0	23	6
Chocolate Roll Icing (1 oz.)	97	0.71	N/A	0	0.28	22	27
Doughnut	340	22	N/A	0	4.5	28	340
Doughnut Glaze (1 oz.)	88	0	N/A	0	0	22	1.4
Boston Market							
Low-fat foods							
Skinless Rotisserie Turkey Breast	170	1	0.5	10	36	1	850
Chicken Sandwich, no cheese or sauce	390	5	1	55	31	60	810
Turkey Sandwich, no cheese or sauce	390	3.5	0.5	60	33	61	1,030
Ham Sandwich, no cheese or sauce	410	8	2.5	45	25	65	1,390
1/4 White Chicken, no skin or wing	170	4	1	85	33	2	480
Fruit Salad	70	0.5	0	0	1	15	10
Red Beans and Rice	260	5	0	5	8	45	1,050
Cranberry Walnut Relish	350	4.5	0	0	3	75	0
Garlic and Dill New Potatoes	130	2.5	0	0	3	25	150
Herb Buttered Corn	180	4	0.5	0	5	30	170
Butternut Squash	150	6	4	20	2	25	560
Steamed Vegetables	35	0.5	0	0	2	7	35
Entrees							
1/4 White Chicken, with skin and wing	280	12	3.5	135	40	2	510
1/4 Dark Chicken, no skin	190	10	3	115	22	1	440
1/4 Dark Chicken, with skin	320	21	6	155	30	2	500
1/2 Chicken, with skin	590	33	10	280	70	4	1,010
Honey Glazed Ham (lean)	210	8	3	75	24	10	1,460
Meatloaf	290	17	8	70	20	15	590

Item	Calories	Fat (g)	Sat. fat (g)	Cholesterol (mg)	Protein (g)	Carbs (g)	Sodium (mg)
1/2 Chicken, with skin	590	33	10	280	70	4	1,010
Meatloaf and Chunky Tomato Sauce	310	17	8	70	21	21	1,010
Meatloaf and Brown Gravy	340	21	8	70	21	18	870
Chicken Pot Pie	750	46	14	110	26	57	1,530
Chunky Chicken Salad	480	39	6	110	25	4	930
Hot sides							
BBQ Baked Beans	270	5	2	0	8	48	540
Black Beans and Rice	300	10	1.5	0	8	45	1,050
Broccoli Rice Casserole	240	12	8	40	5	26	800
Chicken Gravy	15	0.5	0	0	0	2	180
Creamed Spinach	260	20	13	55	9	11	740
Glazed Carrots	280	15	3	0	1	35	80
Green Beans	80	6	1	0	1	5	200
Green Bean Casserole	80	4.5	1.5	5	1	9	670
Homestyle Mashed Potatoes	210	9	5	25	4	30	590
Homestyle Mashed Potatoes and Gravy	230	9	5	25	4	32	780
Hot Cinnamon Apples	250	4.5	0.5	0	0	56	45
Macaroni and Cheese	280	11	6	30	13	33	890
Rice Pilaf	180	5	1	0	5	32	600
Savory Stuffing	310	12	2	0	6	44	1,140
Squash Casserole	330	24	13	70	7	20	1,110
Sweet Potato Casserole	280	18	4.5	10	3	39	190
Cold sides							
Caesar Side Salad	200	17	4.5	15	7	7	450
Coleslaw	300	19	3	20	2	30	540
Cucumber Salad	120	10	1.5	0	2	9	900
Tortellini Salad	350	24	6	55	11	24	530
Jumpin' Juice Squares	150	0	0	0	4	32	140
Old-Fashioned Potato Salad	200	12	2	15	3	22	450
Sandwiches							
Chicken Sandwich, with cheese and sauce	630	28	8	90	37	61	930
Chicken Salad Sandwich	680	30	5	120	39	63	1,360
Turkey Sandwich, with cheese and sauce	620	25	7	110	39	64	1,300
Ham Sandwich, with cheese and sauce	650	31	9	85	31	67	1,730
Meatloaf Sandwich, with cheese	690	27	12	90	36	83	1,480

Item	Calories	Fat (g)	Sat. fat (g)	Cholesterol (mg)	Protein (g)	Carbs (g)	Sodium (mg)
Sandwiches (continued)							
Open-Faced Meatloaf Sandwich	730	36	14	95	29	74	2,180
Turkey Bacon Club Sandwich	780	38	14	145	47	64	1,800
Open-Faced Turkey Sandwich	720	20	7	105	41	93	2,850
BBQ Chicken Sandwich	540	9	2.5	75	30	84	1,690
Soups and salads							
Caesar Side Salad	470	39	7	25	11	20	1,040
Caesar Salad Entree	670	57	11	40	18	24	1,480
Caesar Salad, no dressing	230	12	6	20	16	14	500
Chicken Caesar Salad	810	60	12	105	43	25	1,840
Chicken Caesar Salad, no dressing	390	16	5	80	40	22	880
Chicken Noodle Soup	100	4.5	1.5	30	6	8	500
Chicken Tortilla Soup	170	8	2.5	25	8	18	1,060
Turkey Tortilla Soup	160	7	2	20	9	18	1,090
Baked goods							
Cornbread	200	6	1.5	25	3	33	390
Nestle Toll House Chocolate Chip Cookie	390	19	6	15	4	51	350
Nestle Toll House Oatmeal Scotchie Cookie	390	20	5	30	5	47	340
Nestle Toll House Peanut Butter Chip Cookie	420	25	7	20	7	43	380
Chocolate Brownie	310	10	1	5	3	51	150
Oreo Brownie	560	20	3.5	5	4	90	550
Rice Krispie Treat	420	8	1.5	0	5	83	610
Apple Streusel Pie	480	18	5	15	4	63	105
Cherry Streusel Pie	410	17	5	10	4	60	105
Pecan Pie	550	27	7	110	5	71	100
Pumpkin Pie	370	17	5	50	5	50	60
Cheesecake	580	41	22	165	9	44	400
Chocolate Cake	510	24	6	25	3	73	320
Hummingbird Cake	710	36	14	85	6	92	350
Burger King							
Burgers							
Original Whopper	760	46	14	100	35	52	1,000
Original Whopper, no mayo	600	28	12	85	34	52	870
Original Whopper with Cheese	850	53	30	120	39	53	1,430
Original Whopper with Cheese, no mayo	690	36	17	110	39	53	1,310

Item	Calories	Fat (g)	Sat. fat (g)	Cholesterol (mg)	Protein (g)	Carbs (g)	Sodium (mg)
Original Double Whopper	1,060	69	25	185	59	52	1,100
Original Double Whopper, no mayo	900	51	22	175	59	52	980
Original Double Whopper with Cheese	1,150	76	30	210	64	53	1,530
Original Double Whopper with Cheese, no mayo	990	59	28	195	64	53	1,410
Original Whopper Jr.	390	22	7	45	17	32	570
Original Whopper Jr., no mayo	310	13	5	40	17	31	510
Original Whopper Jr. with Cheese	440	26	9	55	19	32	790
Original Whopper Jr. with Cheese, no mayo	360	17	8	50	19	32	730
BK Homestyle Griller	480	27	11	75	26	35	760
BK Smokehouse Cheddar Griller	720	48	19	125	39	32	1,240
King Supreme Sandwich	550	34	14	100	30	32	790
BK 1/4 Lb. Burger	490	21	8	60	26	50	950
Hamburger	310	13	5	40	17	31	580
Cheeseburger	360	17	8	50	19	31	790
Double Hamburger	450	24	10	75	28	31	620
Double Cheeseburger	540	31	15	100	32	32	1,050
Bacon Double Cheeseburger	580	34	17	110	35	32	1,240
Sandwiches and sides							
BK Big Fish Sandwich	710	39	15	50	24	68	1,160
Chicken Whopper	580	26	5	75	39	48	1,370
Chicken Whopper, no mayo	420	9	2.5	60	38	47	1,250
Chicken Whopper Jr.	350	14	2.5	45	26	30	900
Chicken Whopper Jr., no mayo	270	6	1.5	40	25	30	840
Specialty Chicken Sandwich	560	28	6	60	25	52	1,270
Specialty Chicken Sandwich, no mayo	460	17	4.5	55	25	52	1,190
Chicken Tenders							
4 Pieces	170	9	2.5	25	11	10	420
5 Pieces	210	12	3.5	30	14	13	530
6 Pieces	250	14	4	35	16	15	630
8 Pieces	340	19	5	50	22	20	840

Item	Calories	Fat (g)	Sat. fat (g)	Cholesterol (mg)	Protein (g)	Carbs (g)	Sodium (mg)
BK Veggie Burger	330	10	1.5	0	14	45	770
BK Veggie Burger, no mayo	290	7	1	0	14	44	690
French fries							
Small (salted)	230	11	3	0	3	29	410
Small (no salt added)	230	11	3	0	3	29	240
Medium (salted)	360	18	5	0	4	46	640
Medium (no salt added)	360	18	5	0	4	46	380
Large (salted)	500	25	7	0	6	63	880
Large (no salt added)	500	25	7	0	6	63	510
King (salted)	600	30	8	0	7	76	1,070
King (no salt added)	600	30	8	0	7	76	620
Onion rings							
Small	180	9	2	0	2	22	260
Medium	320	16	4	0	4	40	460
Large	480	23	6	0	7	60	690
King	550	27	7	5	8	70	800
Salads							
Chicken Caesar (no dressing or croutons)	160	6	3	40	25	5	730
Garden Salad (no dressing)	25	0	0	0	1	5	15
Desserts							
Dutch Apple Pie	340	14	3	1	2	52	470
Hershey's Sundae Pie	310	18	13	10	3	33	135
Hot Fudge Brownie Royale	440	19	6	50	6	62	250
French Baked Cookies	440	21	7	15	4	57	390
Breakfast							
Croissan'Wich with Sausage, Egg, & Cheese	520	39	14	210	19	24	1,090
Croissan'Wich with Sausage & Cheese	420	31	11	45	14	23	840
Croissan'Wich with Egg & Cheese	320	19	7	185	12	24	730
Egg'Wich with Canadian Bacon, Egg, & Cheese	420	23	7	140	18	36	900
Egg'Wich with Canadian Bacon & Egg	380	19	4	125	15	35	680
Egg'Wich with Egg & Cheese	410	23	7	130	15	36	760
French Toast Sticks, 5 sticks	390	20	4.5	0	6	46	440
Cini-mini (no vanilla icing), 4 rolls	440	23	6	25	6	51	710

Item	Calories	Fat (g)	Sat. fat (g)	Cholesterol (mg)	Protein (g)	Carbs (g)	Sodium (mg)
Hash Brown Rounds							
Small	230	15	4	0	2	23	450
Large	390	25	7	0	3	38	760
Beverages							
Old-Fashioned Ice Cream Shakes							
Vanilla, small	560	32	21	95	11	56	220
Vanilla, medium	720	41	27	125	15	73	280
Chocolate, small	620	32	21	95	12	72	310
Chocolate, medium	790	42	27	125	15	89	380
Strawberry, small	620	32	21	95	11	71	230
Strawberry, medium	780	41	27	125	15	88	300
Minute Maid Orange Juice	140	0	0	0	0	33	25
Coffee							
Small	0	0	0	0	0	< 1	0
Medium	5	0	0	0	0	< 1	5
Large	10	0	0	0	0	2	10
1% Milk (8 fl. oz.)	110	2.5	1.5	10	8	12	125
Original Whopper patty	320	23	11	85	25	0	100
Original Whopper bun	260	5	1	0	9	45	390
Hamburger patty	140	10	4.5	40	11	0	45
Hamburger bun	160	3	0.5	0	5	28	280
BK Back Porch Griller patty	160	13	5	40	10	1	80
BK Homestyle bun	140	1	0	0	6	29	270
Breaded chicken patty	240	13	4	55	18	13	790
Chicken Sandwich bun	210	3.5	0.5	0	7	39	390
Chicken Whopper patty	160	4	1	75	28	3	1,080
Chicken Whopper Jr. patty	100	2.5	0.5	50	18	2	710
Fish patty	220	9	1.5	35	15	20	460
BK Veggie patty	120	4	0.5	0	8	14	410
Creamy Smokehouse Sauce (1/2 oz.)	70	7	1	5	0	1	90
King Supreme Sauce (1/2 oz.)	70	7	1	10	0	2	105
Ketchup (1/2 oz.)	15	0	0	0	0	4	180
Lettuce (3/4 oz.)	5	0	0	0	0	0	0
Mayonnaise (3/4 oz.)	160	17	2.5	10	0	0	125
Reduced-fat mayonnaise (3/8 oz.)	70	6	1	0	0	3	160
Mustard (1/9 oz.)	5	0	0	0	0	0	40
Onion (1/2 oz.)	5	0	0	0	0	1	0
Pickles (4 slices)	0	0	0	0	0	0	200

Item	Calories	Fat (g)	Sat. fat (g)	Cholesterol (mg)	Protein (g)	Carbs (g)	Sodium (mg)
Processed American cheese (2 slices)	90	8	5	20	5	1	440
Smoked natural white cheddar cheese (1 slice)	90	7	4	20	5	0	135
Tartar sauce (1/2 oz.)	80	8	4	5	0	0	105
Tomato (2 slices)	5	0	0	0	0	1	0
Breakfast components							
Bacon (3 half slices)	40	3	1	10	3	0	210
Canadian bacon (1 slice)	15	0	0	10	3	0	140
Puffed scrambled egg portion	100	8	2.5	170	5	2	250
Fried egg patty	90	7	1.5	120	6	1	140
Ham (2 slices)	35	1	0	15	6	0	780
Sausage patty (2 oz.)	260	25	8	35	9	0	450
Croissant	170	7	2	5	5	22	270
English muffin	210	5	1	0	7	34	340
Grape jam	30	0	0	0	0	7	0
Strawberry jam	30	0	0	0	0	7	0
Breakfast syrup	80	0	0	0	0	21	20
Vanilla icing (Cini-minis)	110	3	0.5	0	0	20	40
Dipping sauces							
Barbecue Dipping Sauce	35	0	0	0	0	9	390
Honey Flavored Dipping Sauce	90	0	0	0	0	23	0
Honey Mustard Dipping Sauce	90	6	1	10	0	9	150
Sweet and Sour Dipping Sauce	40	0	0	0	0	10	65
Ranch Dipping Sauce	140	15	2.5	5	1	1	95
Zesty Onion Ring Dipping Sauce	150	15	2.5	15	0	3	210
Salad dressings and toppings							
Kraft Catalina Dressing	180	16	2.5	0	0	10	530
Signature Creamy Caesar Dressing	140	13	2	10	1	4	340
Kraft Ranch Dressing	220	23	3.5	10	0	2	410
Kraft Thousand Island Dressing	110	9	1.5	10	1	7	410
Light Done Right Light Italian Dressing	50	4.5	0.5	0	0	4	360
Croutons (3/4 oz.)	90	3	0	0	2	14	300
Parmesan cheese (1/2 oz.)	45	3.5	2	0	4	0	170

Item	Calories	Fat (g)	Sat. fat (g)	Cholesterol (mg)	Protein (g)	Carbs (g)	Sodium (mg)
Carl's Jr.							
Sandwiches							
Carl's Famous Star	590	32	9	70	24	50	910
Super Star	790	47	15	130	41	51	980
Sourdough Bacon Cheeseburger	640	41	15	95	30	37	690
Sourdough Ranch Bacon Cheeseburger	720	46	16	95	33	43	800
Double Sourdough Bacon Cheeseburger	880	59	24	165	50	37	1,010
Western Bacon Cheeseburger	660	30	12	85	31	64	1,410
Double Western Bacon Cheeseburger	920	50	21	155	51	65	1,770
Famous Bacon Cheeseburger	700	41	13	95	31	51	1,310
Hamburger	280	9	3.5	35	14	36	480
Charbroiled BBQ Chicken Sandwich	290	3.5	1	60	25	41	840
Charbroiled BBQ Club Sandwich	470	23	7	95	31	37	1,110
Charbroiled Santa Fe Chicken Sandwich	540	31	8	95	28	37	1,210
Carl's Ranch Crispy Chicken Sandwich	660	31	7	70	24	71	1,180
Carl's Bacon Swiss Crispy Chicken Sandwich	760	38	11	90	31	72	1,550
Carl's Western Bacon Crispy Chicken Sandwich	750	28	11	80	31	91	1,900
Spicy Chicken Sandwich	480	26	5	40	14	47	1,220
Southwest Spicy Chicken Sandwich	620	41	10	65	16	48	1,640
Charbroiled Sirloin Steak Sandwich	550	24	4.5	80	30	52	1,080
Carl's Catch Fish Sandwich	530	28	7	80	18	55	1,030
American Cheese, large	60	5	3.5	15	3	1	260
American Cheese, small	50	4	2.5	10	3	1	200
Swiss-Style Cheese	50	4	2.5	15	4	0	230
Sides							
French Fries, kids	250	12	2.5	0	4	32	150
French Fries, small	290	14	3	0	5	37	180
French Fries, medium	460	22	5	0	7	59	280
French Fries, large	620	29	6	0	10	80	380
Onion rings	430	22	5	0	7	53	700

Item	Calories	Fat (g)	Sat. fat (g)	Cholesterol (mg)	Protein (g)	Carbs (g)	Sodium (mg)
Sides (continued)							
Zucchini	320	19	5	0	6	31	860
Hash Brown Nuggets	330	21	4.5	0	3	32	470
CrissCut Fries	410	24	5	0	5	43	950
Chicken Stars (6 pieces)	260	16	4.5	40	13	14	480
Potatoes							
Broccoli and cheese	530	21	5	15	11	76	940
Bacon and cheese	640	29	9	40	21	75	1,660
Plain, no margarine	290	0	0	0	6	68	20
Sour cream and chives	430	14	4	10	7	70	180
Salad							
Charbroiled Chicken Salad-to-go	200	7	3	75	25	12	440
Garden Salad-to-go	50	2.5	1.5	5	3	4	60
Condiments							
House Dressing	220	22	3.5	25	1	3	450
Blue Cheese Dressing	320	35	7	25	2	1	370
Thousand Island Dressing	230	23	4	20	< 1	5	420
Fat-Free Italian Dressing	15	0	0	0	0	4	770
Fat-Free French Dressing	60	0	0	0	0	16	660
Croutons	30	1	0	0	1	5	105
Breadsticks	35	0.5	0	0	1	7	60
Table syrup	90	0	0	0	0	21	0
Salsa	10	0	0	0	0	2	160
Mustard Sauce	50	0	0	0	0	11	210
Honey Sauce	90	0	0	0	0	22	0
BBQ Sauce	50	0	0	0	1	11	270
Sweet n' Sour Sauce	50	0	0	0	0	12	80
Grape jelly	40	0	0	0	0	9	15
Strawberry jam	40	0	0	0	0	9	15
Breakfast							
Sourdough Breakfast	410	20	10	275	26	33	930
Sunrise Sandwich	360	21	8	245	13	28	470
Breakfast Burrito	550	32	11	495	29	36	980
French Toast Dips	370	20	2.5	0	6	42	430
Breakfast Quesadilla	370	17	5	240	16	38	910
Scrambled eggs	180	14	3	455	13	1	110
English Muffin, with margarine	210	9	2	0	5	28	300
Bacon, 2 strips	45	4	1.5	10	3	0	150
Sausage, 1 patty	190	18	6	40	7	2	480
Baked goods							
Blueberry Muffin	340	14	2	40	5	49	340

Item	Calories	Fat (g)	Sat. fat (g)	Cholesterol (mg)	Protein (g)	Carbs (g)	Sodium (mg)
Bran Raisin Muffin	370	14	2	45	6	61	410
Chocolate Chip Cookie	350	18	7	20	3	46	330
Chocolate Cake	300	12	3	30	3	48	350
Cheese Danish	400	23	6	15	5	49	390
Strawberry Swirl Cheesecake	290	17	9	55	6	30	230
Beverages							
Orange juice	150	0	0	0	1	37	0
1% Milk	150	3	2	15	14	18	180
Vanilla shake, small	470	11	7	50	15	78	350
Vanilla shake, regular	700	16	11	70	22	115	530
Chocolate shake, small	530	10	7	45	14	96	350
Chocolate shake, regular	770	15	10	65	21	140	520
Strawberry shake, small	510	10	7	45	14	91	330
Strawberry shake, regular	750	15	10	65	20	133	490
Raspberry Nestea, regular	160	0	0	0	0	42	40
Iced tea	5	0	0	0	0	0	10
Hot chocolate	120	2	2	0	2	22	125
Coffee	2	< 1	0	0	< 1	< 1	< 5
Chick-Fil-A							
Sandwiches							
Chick-Fil-A Chicken Sandwich	410	16	3.5	60	28	38	1,300
Chick-Fil-A Chicken Sandwich, no butter	380	13	3	60	28	37	1,290
Chicken Deluxe Sandwich	420	16	3.5	60	28	39	1,300
Chicken (1 filet, no bun, no pickles)	230	11	2.5	60	23	10	990
Chargrilled chicken sandwiches							
Chick-Fil-A Chargrilled Chicken Sandwich	280	7	2	60	25	29	1,000
Chick-Fil-A Chargrilled Chicken Sandwich, no butter	240	3.5	1	60	25	28	1,000
Chargrilled Chicken Deluxe Sandwich	280	7	2	60	26	30	1,010
Chargrilled Chicken (1 filet, no bun, no pickles)	100	1.5	0	60	20	1	690
Chargrilled Chicken Club Sandwich, no sauce	360	13	5	80	30	31	1,370

Item	Calories	Fat (g)	Sat. fat (g)	Cholesterol (mg)	Protein (g)	Carbs (g)	Sodium (mg)
Cool Wraps							
Chargrilled Chicken Cool Wrap	390	7	3	70	31	53	1,120
Chicken Caesar Cool Wrap	460	11	6	85	38	51	1,540
Spicy Chicken Caesar Cool Wrap	390	7	3.5	70	31	51	1,150
Specialties							
Chick-Fil-A Chick-N-Strips (4)	250	11	2.5	70	25	12	570
Chick-Fil-A Nuggets (8)	260	12	2.5	70	26	12	1,090
Chick-Fil-A Chicken Salad Sandwich, on whole wheat bread	350	15	3	65	20	32	880
Hearty Breast of Chicken Soup (7.6 oz.)	100	1.5	0	20	9	13	940
Salads							
Chick-Fil-A Chargrilled Chicken Garden Salad	180	6	3	70	23	8	730
Chick-Fil-A Chargrilled Chicken Caesar Salad	240	10	6	85	31	6	1,170
Chick-Fil-A Chick-N-Strips Salad	340	16	5	85	30	19	680
Sides							
Side Salad	80	5	2.5	15	5	6	110
Coleslaw	210	17	2.5	20	1	14	180
Carrot & Raisin Salad (small)	130	5	1	0	1	22	90
Chick-Fil-A Waffle Potato Fries (small, salted)	280	14	5	15	3	37	105
Chick-Fil-A Waffle Potato Fries (small, unsalted)	280	14	5	15	3	36	40
Condiments							
Polynesian Sauce	110	6	1	0	0	13	210
Dijon Honey Mustard Sauce	50	5	0.5	5	0	2	65
Barbecue Sauce	45	0	0	0	0	11	180
Honey Mustard Sauce	45	0	0	0	0	10	150
Caesar Dressing	200	21	3.5	45	1	1	300
Basil Vinaigrette Dressing	210	21	3.5	0	0	4	160
Blue Cheese Dressing	190	20	4	20	1	2	370
Buttermilk Ranch Dressing	190	20	3	10	1	2	330
Spicy Dressing	210	22	3.5	10	0	2	170

Item	Calories	Fat (g)	Sat. fat (g)	Cholesterol (mg)	Protein (g)	Carbs (g)	Sodium (mg)
Thousand Island Dressing	170	16	2.5	10	0	6	300
Truett's Special House Dressing	150	13	2	5	0	7	290
Light Italian Dressing	20	0.5	0	0	0	3	640
Fat-Free Dijon Honey Mustard Dressing	60	0	0	0	0	14	200
Garlic and Butter Croutons	90	4	0	0	2	11	140
Roasted sunflower kernels (unsalted)	80	7	1	0	3	3	0
Desserts							
Icedream (small cup)	230	6	3.5	25	5	38	100
Icedream (small cone)	160	4	2	15	4	28	80
Lemon pie	320	10	3.5	110	7	51	220
Fudge Nut Brownie	330	15	3.5	20	4	45	210
Cheesecake	340	21	12	90	6	30	270
Cheesecake, with strawberry topping	360	21	12	90	6	38	290
Cheesecake, with blueberry topping	370	21	12	90	6	39	280
Del Taco							
Burritos							
Macho Beef Burrito	1,170	62	29	190	60	89	2,190
Macho Chicken Burrito	930	33	15	100	47	111	2,990
Macho Combo Burrito	1,050	44	21	115	49	113	2,760
Deluxe Del Beef Burrito	590	33	19	95	32	45	1,110
Del Beef Burrito	550	30	17	90	31	42	1,090
Deluxe Combo Burrito	570	25	15	60	29	64	1,700
Del Combo Burrito	530	22	13	55	28	61	1,680
Del Classic Chicken Burrito	560	36	13	70	24	41	1,100
Spicy Chicken Burrito	480	16	10	40	23	66	1,850
Veggie Works Burrito	490	18	11	25	18	69	1,660
Chicken Works Burrito	520	23	12	65	26	57	1,620
Steak Works Burrito	590	31	16	70	27	58	1,820
Half Pound Red Burrito	430	12	9	20	20	65	1,670
Half Pound Green Burrito	430	12	9	20	20	59	1,690
Bean & Cheese Red Burrito	270	8	5	15	11	38	1,020
Bean & Cheese Green Burrito	280	8	5	15	11	38	1,030
Quesadillas							
Chicken	580	31	21	104	33	41	1,240
Spicy Jack Chicken	570	30	16	105	32	40	1,300

Item	Calories	Fat (g)	Sat. fat (g)	Cholesterol (mg)	Protein (g)	Carbs (g)	Sodium (mg)
Quesadillas (continued)							
Regular	500	27	20	75	23	39	860
Spicy Jack	490	26	17	75	23	38	920
Salads							
Deluxe Taco Salad	780	40	18	80	33	76	2,250
Deluxe Chicken Salad	740	34	15	70	33	77	2,610
Taco Salad	350	30	10	45	10	10	390
Chicken Fiesta Bowl, with ancho chile sauce	550	27	5	80	27	50	2,210
Chicken Fiesta Bowl, no ancho chile sauce	420	13	3	60	26	49	2,040
Veggie Fiesta Bowl, with ancho chile sauce	490	22	4	20	10	64	1,830
Sandwiches							
Double Del Cheeseburger	560	35	12	85	26	35	960
Bacon Double Del Cheeseburger	610	39	14	95	29	35	1,130
Del Cheeseburger	430	25	7	45	16	35	710
Cheeseburger	330	13	6	35	16	37	870
Hamburger	280	9	3	25	13	37	640
Bun Taco	440	21	12	65	24	37	830
Tacos							
Big Fat Steak Taco	390	19	6	45	18	38	960
Big Fat Chicken Taco	340	13	4	45	18	38	840
Big Fat Taco	320	11	5	35	16	39	680
Big Fat Crispy Chicken Taco	620	38	9	60	21	52	1,070
Sides							
Macho Nachos	1,100	63	24	55	31	113	2,640
Nachos	380	24	8	5	5	40	630
Deluxe Chili Cheese Fries	710	49	16	50	17	53	880
Chili Cheese Fries	670	46	15	45	17	51	880
Macho Fries	690	46	7	0	7	68	550
Large Fries	490	32	5	0	5	47	380
Regular Fries	350	23	4	0	3	34	270
Small Fries	210	14	2	0	2	20	160
Rice Cup	140	2	1	2	3	27	910
Bean 'N Cheese Cup	260	3	2	5	16	44	1,810
Breakfast							
Macho Bacon & Egg Burrito	1,030	60	20	790	40	82	1,760
Steak & Egg Burrito	580	34	16	560	33	41	1,270
Egg & Cheese Burrito	450	24	13	530	23	39	740

Item	Calories	Fat (g)	Sat. fat (g)	Cholesterol (mg)	Protein (g)	Carbs (g)	Sodium (mg)
Breakfast Burrito	250	11	6	160	10	24	520
Bacon & Egg Quesadilla	450	23	12	260	21	40	920
Bacon, 2 slices	50	4	1.5	10	3	0	170
Beverages							
Chocolate shake, small	520	12	9	35	12	89	270
Chocolate shake, large	680	16	12	45	16	117	350
Strawberry shake, small	410	6	4	30	11	76	220
Strawberry shake, large	540	8	6	40	14	100	280
Vanilla shake, small	420	7	5	35	12	75	250
Vanilla shake, large	550	10	6	50	16	97	320
Domino's Pizza							
6" Deep Dish Cheese Pizza	598	28	10	36	23	68	1,341
12" Medium Cheese Pizza, 2 slices							
Hand-Tossed	374	11	5	23	15	55	776
Thin Crust	273	12	5	23	12	31	835
Deep Dish	482	22	8	30	19	56	1,123
Medium combinations (add to preceding values)							
Pepperoni	147	13	6	32	8	1	527
Vegi	65	5	2	11	4	3	211
America's Favorite	135	11	5	29	7	3	450
Hawaiian	76	5	2	18	6	4	326
Meatzza	185	15	7	42	11	2	687
Deluxe	90	7	3	17	4	3	287
Extravaganzza	153	12	5	30	8	3	573
14" Large Cheese Pizza, 2 slices							
Hand-Tossed	516	15	7	32	21	75	1,080
Thin Crust	382	17	7	32	17	43	1,171
Deep Dish	677	30	11	41	26	80	1,576
Large combinations (add to preceding values)							
Pepperoni	203	17	8	44	11	2	729
Vegi	89	7	3	16	5	3	289
America's Favorite	175	14	7	37	10	3	580
Hawaiian	107	6	3	26	8	5	463
Meatzza	237	19	9	53	14	3	867
Deluxe	112	9	4	21	5	3	352
Extravaganzza	189	15	6	37	10	4	700
Sides							
Barbecue Wings (1)	50	2	0.7	26	6	2	175
Hot Wings (1)	45	2	0.07	26	6	1	354
Breadsticks (1)	116	4	1	0	3	18	152
Cheesy Bread (1)	142	6	2	6	4	18	183

Item	Calories	Fat (g)	Sat. fat (g)	Cholesterol (mg)	Protein (g)	Carbs (g)	Sodium (mg)
El Pollo Loco							
Bowls							
Pollo Choice Skinless Breast Bowl	340	15	N/A	110	38	16	925
Pollo Bowl	469	11	2	42	30	66	1868
Smokey Black Bean Bowl	604	23	7	54	29	75	1955
Flame Broiled Chicken Bowl	357	13	2	42	25	39	1079
Mexican Chicken Salad Bowl	494	30	6	55	26	32	1175
Nacho Pollo Bowl	766	33	10	87	37	64	1358
Burritos							
Ultimate	633	23	8	89	39	66	1237
Mexican Chicken Caesar	734	35	8	49	36	65	1214
Spicy	633	21	8	69	31	80	1495
Chicken Lover's	479	19	6	143	29	47	1373
Ranch	616	30	13	127	40	45	1356
Classic	580	22	7	108	31	66	1595
BRC	503	16	6	17	17	73	1263
Flame-broiled Chicken							
Breast	160	6	2	110	26	0	390
Leg	90	5	1.5	75	11	0	150
Thigh	180	12	4	130	16	0	230
Wing	110	6	2	80	12	0	220
Miscellaneous							
Chicken Sticks (Kids)	226	12	1.3	53	17	15	787
Chicken Quesadilla	593	29	12	107	36	48	1329
Chicken Nachos	1420	92	26	161	47	105	1506
Chicken Tostado Salad	990	52	12	82	39	62	1755
Barbecue Chicken Tostada Salad (w/o shell & sour cream)	543	24	3	55	27	55	1650
Tostado Shell only	440	27	4	25	15	43	690
Chicken Taquito	370	17	4	25	15	43	690
Chicken Tamale	180	8	1.5	15	7	21	490
Tacos							
Taco al Carbon	180	8	1	19	7	20	152
Chicken Soft Taco	237	12	4	74	17	15	629
Sides (individual)							
Coleslaw	206	16	3	11	2	12	358
Corn Cobbette 3"	80	1	0	0	3	18	10
Mashed Potatoes	97	1	0	0	3	21	369
Gravy	13	0.5	0	1	0.4	2	.2
Pinto Beans	185	4	0	0	11	29	744

Item	Calories	Fat (g)	Sat. fat (g)	Cholesterol (mg)	Protein (g)	Carbs (g)	Sodium (mg)
Potato Salad	256	14	2	15	527	3	30
Smokey Black Beans	306	16	6	13	7	35	731
Spanish Rice	130	3	1	0	2	24	397
Garden Salad	105	7	3	15	5	7	99
Macaroni & Cheese	244	12	4	22	10	24	950
Fresh Vegetables	57	2	0.5	0	2	8	79
Tortilla Chips, unsalted	426	24	5	0	5	48	12
Tortillas							
4.5" Corn	32	0.5	0	0	1	6	21
6" Corn	70	1	0	0	1	14	35
6.5" Flour	110	4	0	0	3	13	16
11" Flour	260	7	2	0	7	42	583
Spicy Tomato	254	6	1	0	7	42	577
Dressings							
Light Italian	20	1	0	0	0	2	780
Ranch	220	24	4	10	1	2	420
1,000 Island	220	21	3	30	0	7	360
Bleu Cheese	230	24	5	30	2	2	450
Creamy Cilantro	266	29	4	13	1	1	306
Hidden Valley Ranch	110	11	1.5	10	1	1	250
Condiments							
Guacamole	30	2	0	0	0	3	160
Jalapeno Hot Sauce	5	0	0	0	0	1	110
Sour cream	60	5	3.5		1	1	15
House salsa	6	0	0	0	0	1	96
Pico de Gallo salsa	11	0.5	0	0	0	1.5	131
Spicy Chipotle salsa	7	0	0	0	0	1	180
Avocado salsa	12	1	0	0	0	1	204
Desserts							
Churros	179	11	3	5	3	18	221
Foster's Freeze (w/o cone)	180	5	3	20	4	30	100
Berry Banana Smoothie	367	7	3	23	3	68	136
Kiwi Strawberry Smoothie	357	7	3	23	5	66	141
Banana Split	717	28	11	56	12	107	31
Hardee's							
Breakfast							
Scratch Biscuit	390	21	6	0	6	44	1000
Jelly Biscuit	440	21	6	0	6	57	1000
Apple Cinnamon 'N' Raisin Biscuit	250	8	2	0	2	42	350
Sausage Biscuit	550	36	11	25	12	44	1310
Sausage & Egg Biscuit	620	41	13	225	19	45	1370

Item	Calories	Fat (g)	Sat. fat (g)	Cholesterol (mg)	Protein (g)	Carbs (g)	Sodium (mg)
Breakfast (continued)							
Bacon, Egg & Cheese Biscuit	520	30	11	210	17	45	1420
Country Ham Biscuit	440	22	7	30	14	44	1710
Frisco Breakfast Sandwich (ham)	450	22	8	225	22	42	1290
Ham Biscuit	410	20	6	25	13	45	1200
Regular Hash Rounds	230	14	3	0	24	3	560
Biscuit 'N' Gravy	530	30	9	15	10	56	1550
Omelet Biscuit	550	32	12	225	20	45	1350
Chicken Biscuit	590	27	7	45	24	62	1820
Steak Biscuit	580	32	10	30	15	56	1580
Burgers & Sandwiches							
Famous Star	570	35	10	80	24	41	860
Six Dollar Burger	949	62	25	137	38	58	1685
Super Star	790	53	17	145	40	41	970
All-Star	680	43	14	100	29	41	1260
Frisco Burger	720	49	15	95	31	37	1180
Monster Burger	1060	79	29	185	49	37	1860
Hamburger	270	11	4	35	13	29	550
Chicken Fillet Sandwich	480	23	4	55	14	44	1190
Grilled Chicken Sandwich	350	16	3	65	23	28	860
Bacon Swiss Crispy chicken	670	44	9	55	24	45	1600
Regular Roast Beef	310	16	6	40	17	26	800
Big Roast Beef Sandwich	410	24	9	40	24	26	1140
Monster Roast Beef	610	39	18	105	35	26	1940
Hot Ham 'N Cheese Sandwich	300	12	6	50	16	34	1390
Fisherman's Fillet Sandwich	530	28	7	75	25	45	1280
Hot Dog (w/ condiments)	450	32	12	55	15	25	1240
Chicken							
Breast	370	15	4	75	29	29	1190
Wing	200	8	2	30	10	23	740
Thigh	330	15	4	60	19	30	1000
Leg	170	7	2	45	13	15	570
Sides							
Coleslaw (small)	240	20	3	10	2	13	340
Gravy	20	<1	<1	0	<1	3	260
Mashed Potatoes (small)	70	<1	<1	0	2	14	330
Peach Cobbler	310	7	1	0	2	60	360
French Fries							
Regular	340	16	2	0	4	45	390

Item	Calories	Fat (g)	Sat. fat (g)	Cholesterol (mg)	Protein (g)	Carbs (g)	Sodium (mg)
Large	440	21	3	0	5	59	520
Monster	510	24	3	0	6	67	590
Crispy Curls							
Medium	340	18	4	0	5	41	950
Large	520	28	5	0	7	62	1450
Monster	590	31	6	0	8	70	1640
Desserts							
Vanilla Shake	350	5	3	20	12	65	300
Chocolate Shake	370	5	3	30	13	67	270
Twist Cone	160	2	1	10	4	34	120
Apple Turnover	270	12	4	0	4	38	250
In-N-Out							
Burgers							
Hamburger	390	19	5	40	16	39	640
Hamburger w/mustard & ketchup instead of spread	310	10	4	35	16	41	720
Hamburger, Protein Style	240	17	4.5	40	12	10	370
Cheeseburger	480	27	10	60	22	39	1000
Cheeseburger, w/mustard & ketchup instead of spread	400	18	9	55	22	41	1080
Cheeseburger, Protein Style	330	25	9	60	18	11	720
Double-Double	670	41	18	120	37	40	1430
Double-Double w/mustard & ketchup instead of spread	590	32	17	115	37	42	1510
Double-Double, Protein Style	520	39	17	120	33	11	116
Sides							
French Fries	400	18	5	0	7	54	245
Beverages							
Chocolate Shake	690	36	24	95	9	83	350
Vanilla Shake	680	37	25	90	9	78	390
Strawberry Shake	690	33	22	85	8	91	280
Jack in the Box							
Burgers							
Hamburger	250	9	3.5	30	12	30	610
Hamburger w/cheese	300	13	6	40	14	31	840
Double Cheeseburger	410	22	11	70	20	32	920
Bacon Bacon Cheeseburger	910	59	19	100	38	58	1780
Bacon Ultimate Cheeseburger	1120	75	28	160	52	59	2260
Big Cheeseburger	700	40	16	70	26	59	1340

Item	Calories	Fat (g)	Sat. fat (g)	Cholesterol (mg)	Protein (g)	Carbs (g)	Sodium (mg)
Burgers (continued)							
Big Texax Cheeseburger	610	32	15	65	26	55	1280
Jack's Western Cheeseburger	660	37	14	60	24	59	1100
Jumbo Jack	600	31	11	45	22	12	58
Jumbo Jack w/cheese	690	38	16	75	26	12	60
Sourdough Jack	700	49	16	80	30	36	1220
Ultimate Cheeseburger	990	66	28	130	41	59	1620
Chicken & Fish							
Chicken Breast Pieces (5)	360	17	3	80	27	24	970
Chicken Fajita Pita	330	11	4.5	55	24	35	940
Chicken Sandwich Supreme	410	21	4.5	35	15	39	740
Chicken Supreme	710	39	11	70	30	62	1440
Chicken Teriyaki Bowl	550	3	0.5	35	26	103	1720
Fish & Chips	610	31	7	40	18	66	1240
Grilled Chicken Fillet	430	22	6	60	23	34	910
Jack's Spicy Chicken	650	31	6	60	26	67	1190
Sourdough Grilled Chicken Club	520	28	6	85	33	33	1330
Tacos & Snacks							
Bacon Cheddar Potato Wedges	770	53	16	45	21	52	1330
Cheese sticks (3)	240	12	5	25	11	21	420
Cheese sticks (5)	400	21	8	40	18	35	700
Chili Cheese Curly Fries	630	40	11	30	13	54	1640
Egg Rolls (1)	130	6	2	5	5	15	310
Egg Rolls (3)	400	19	6	15	14	44	920
French Fries							
Regular	330	16	3.5	0	3	44	550
Jumbo	410	20	4.5	0	4	55	690
Super Scoop	580	28	6	0	6	77	960
Monster Taco	280	17	6	35	10	22	560
Onion Rings	500	30	5	0	6	51	420
Seasoned Curly Fries	400	23	5	0	6	45	890
Side Salad	50	3	1.5	10	3	5	65
Stuffed Jalapenos (3)	230	13	6	20	7	22	690
Stuffed Jalapenos (7)	530	30	13	45	15	51	1600
Taco	180	10	3.5	20	7	16	310
Tacquitos (3)	320	17	7	40	14	28	440
Tacquitos (5)	480	24	9	50	19	47	350
Breakfast							
Bacon	20	1.5	0.5	5	2	0	95
Breakfast Jack	310	14	5	210	14	34	770

Item	Calories	Fat (g)	Sat. fat (g)	Cholesterol (mg)	Protein (g)	Carbs (g)	Sodium (mg)
Extreme Sausage Sandwich	720	53	18	280	26	35	1180
French Toast Sticks (4)	430	18	4	10	8	57	460
Hash Brown	150	10	2.5	0	1	2	230
Sausage Biscuit	380	27	8	35	11	25	730
Sausage Croissant	680	50	15	250	18	41	760
Sausage, Egg & Cheese Biscuit	760	60	20	280	25	33	1390
Supreme Croissant	570	37	9	240	19	41	1040
Ultimate Breakfast Sandwich	730	40	11	440	30	66	1870
Shakes & Desserts							
Apple Turnover	320	16	4	0	3	41	370
Cheesecake	310	16	9	55	7	34	220
Double Fudge Cake	310	11	3	25	3	49	270
Ice Cream Shakes (16 oz)							
Cappucino	640	28	18	110	10	85	220
Chocolate	660	29	18	110	11	89	270
Oreo	670	33	19	110	11	81	350
Strawberry	640	28	18	110	10	84	220
Vanilla	570	29	18	115	12	65	220
Sauces & Dressings							
Barbecue Dipping Sauce	45	0	0	0	1	11	330
Blue Cheese Dressing	260	26	4.5	30	1	5	670
Buttermilk House Dipping Sauce	130	13	2	10	0	3	210
Buttermilk House Dressing	310	33	5	20	1	3	470
Frank's Red Hot Buffalo Dipping Sauce	10	0	0	0	0	2	840
Low Calorie Italian Dressing	15	0	0	0	0	4	510
Marinara Sauce	15	0	0	0	0	3	210
Soy Sauce	5	0	0	0	0	1	480
Sweet & Sour Dipping Sauce	45	0	0	0	0	11	160
Taco Sauce	0	0	0	0	0	0	80
Tartar Sauce	210	22	3.5	20	0	2	370
Thousand Island Dressing	160	12	2	15	1	12	490
Condiments							
Croutons	60	1.5	0	0	2	1	130
Guacamole	90	7	2	0	1	5	240
Sauces & Dressings							
Salsa	10	0	0	0	0	2	220
Sour Cream	60	5	3	15	1	2	20

Item	Calories	Fat (g)	Sat. fat (g)	Cholesterol (mg)	Protein (g)	Carbs (g)	Sodium (mg)
Sauces & Dressings (continued)							
Sour Cream	60	5	3	15	1	2	20
Syrup	130	0	0	0	0	32	30
Jamba Juice							
Smoothies (24 oz)							
Aloha Pineapple	470	1.5	N/A	N/A	7	89	N/A
Banana Berry	470	1.5	N/A	N/A	5	112	N/A
Berry Lime Sublime	450	2	N/A	N/A	3	104	N/A
Caribbean Passion	440	2	N/A	N/A	4	102	N/A
Chocolate Moo'd	690	8	N/A	N/A	16	141	N/A
Citrus Squeeze	450	2	N/A	N/A	4	93	N/A
Coldbuster	430	2.5	N/A	N/A	5	100	N/A
Cranberry Craze	420	2	N/A	N/A	6	97	N/A
Jamba Powerboost	440	1.5	N/A	N/A	6	103	N/A
Kiwi Berry Burner	470	0	N/A	N/A	4	112	N/A
Mango-a-Go-Go	500	2	N/A	N/A	4	117	N/A
Nog Nog	650	2.5	N/A	N/A	18	135	N/A
Orange Berry Blitz	410	2.5	N/A	N/A	5	94	N/A
Orange Dream Machine	540	2.5	N/A	N/A	18	112	N/A
Orange-a-Peel	440	1	N/A	N/A	9	102	N/A
Peach Pleasure	460	2	N/A	N/A	4	108	N/A
Peanut Butter Moo'd	840	22	N/A	N/A	23	139	N/A
Peenya Kowlada	650	5	N/A	N/A	8	118	N/A
Protein Berry Pizazz	440	1.5	N/A	N/A	21	102	N/A
Razzmatazz	480	2	N/A	N/A	3	112	N/A
Strawberries Wild	450	0	N/A	N/A	6	105	N/A
KFC							
Chicken							
Original Recipe							
Whole Wing	140	10	2.5	55	9	5	414
Breast	400	24	6	135	29	16	1116
Drumstick	140	9	12	75	13	4	422
Thigh	250	18	4.5	95	16	6	747
Extra Crispy							
Whole Wing	220	15	4	55	10	10	415
Breast	470	28	8	160	39	17	874
Drumstick	195	12	3	77	15	7	375
Thigh	380	27	7	118	21	14	625
Hot & Spicy							
Whole Wing	210	25	4	55	10	9	350
Breast	505	29	8	162	38	23	1170
Drumstick	175	10	3	77	13	9	360
Thigh	355	26	7	126	19	13	630

Item	Calories	Fat (g)	Sat. fat (g)	Cholesterol (mg)	Protein (g)	Carbs (g)	Sodium (mg)
Crispy Strips							
Colonels Crispy Strips (3)	300	16	4	56	26	18	1165
Spicy Crispy Strips (3)	335	15	4	70	25	23	1140
Honey BBQ Strips (3)	377	15	4	45	27	33	1709
Popcorn Chicken							
Small	362	23	6	43	17	21	610
Large	620	40	10	73	30	36	1046
Wings							
Hot Wings (6)	471	33	8	150	27	19	1230
Honey BBQ (6)	607	38	10	193	33	33	1145
Sandwiches							
Original Recipe w/sauce	450	22	5	70	29	33	940
Original Recipe w/o sauce	360	13	3.5	60	29	21	890
Triple Crunch w/sauce	490	29	6	70	28	39	710
Triple Crunch w/o sauce	390	15	4.5	50	25	29	650
Triple Crunch Zinger w/sauce	550	32	7	85	28	39	830
Triple Crunch Zinger w/osauce	390	15	4.5	50	25	36	650
Tender Roast w/sauce	350	15	3	75	32	26	880
Tender Roast w/o sauce	270	5	1.5	65	31	23	690
Honey BBQ	310	6	2	125	28	37	560
Twister	600	34	7	50	22	52	1430
Crispy Caesar Twister	744	41	9	55	27	66	1616
Honey BBQ Crunch Melt	556	26	5	60	33	48	1010
Pot Pie							
Chunky Chicken Pot Pie	770	42	13	70	29	69	2160
Sides							
Mashed Potatoes w/Gravy	120	6	1	<1	1	17	440
Potato wedges	280	13	4	5	5	28	750
Macaroni & Cheese	180	8	3	10	7	21	860
Corn on the Cob	150	1.5	0	0	5	35	20
BBQ Baked Beans	190	3	1	5	6	33	760
Coleslaw	232	13.5	2	8	2	26	284
Green Beans	45	1.5	0.5	5	1	7	730
Mean Greens	70	3	1	10	4	11	650
Biscuit (1)	180	10	2.5	0	4	20	560
Desserts							
Double Choc Chip Cake	320	16	4	55	4	41	230
Little Bucket Parfait:							
Fudge Brownie	280	10	3.5	45	3	44	190
Lemon Creme	410	14	8	20	7	62	290
Chocolate Cream	290	15	11	15	3	37	330

Item	Calories	Fat (g)	Sat. fat (g)	Cholesterol (mg)	Protein (g)	Carbs (g)	Sodium (mg)
Desserts (continued)							
Strawberry Shortcake	200	7	6	10	1	33	220
Colonel's Pies:							
Pecan Pie slice	490	23	5	65	5	66	510
Apple Pie slice	310	14	3	0	2	44	280
Strawberry Creme Pie slice	280	15	8	15	4	32	130
Koo Koo Roo							
Original Skinless Flame Broiled Chicken							
3-piece Original Dark	260	15	4	108	30	0	107
Original Breast & Wing (wing portion contains skin)	212	8	2	135	34	0.7	443
1 Original Breast	155	4	1	97	28	0.3	350
Half Original Chicken (wing portion contains skin)	391	16	4	81	55	6	859
Rotisserie Chicken							
Rotisserie Leg & Thigh	300	18	5	114	31	1	513
Rotisserie Breast & Wing	355	16	4	140	49	1	675
Half Rotisserie Chicken	655	34	9	254	80	2	1188
Fresh Roasted Carved Turkey							
1/4 lb. White meat	153	1	0	95	34	0	59
1/4 lb. Dark meat	212	8	3	96	32	0	89
Hand Carved Turkey Dinner (mashed potatoes, stuffing, gravy, steamed veg., and cranberry sauce)	881	36	13	150	56	83	4529
Turkey Pot Pie	905	45	12	165	42	83	1381
Sandwiches							
Open-faced Turkey Sandwich (mashed potatoes, stuffing, gravy, and cranberry sauce)	761	35	13	150	51	59	4313
Original Chicken Breast Sandwich w/Original sandwich dressing	654	27	5	91	40	64	1206
BBQ Chicken Breast Sandwich w/ BBQ sauce	497	16	7	135	44	46	1548
Chicken Caesar Sandwich w/Caesar Dressing	791	36	13	137	56	65	2073
Turkey Breast Sandwich w/lite mayo	538	24	6	168	48	31	789
1/2 Turkey Breast Sandwich w/lite mayo	271	12	3	58	24	16	406

Item	Calories	Fat (g)	Sat. fat (g)	Cholesterol (mg)	Protein (g)	Carbs (g)	Sodium (mg)
Bowls and Wings							
Chargrilled Chicken Chop (w/o sauce)	582	11	4.5	133	52	66	670
Southwestern Chicken Chop (w/o sauce)	635	11	4	125	60	79	1404
6 Buffalo Wings	565	27	7	113	40	35	1189
9 Buffalo Wings	848	41	11	170	60	53	1783
Salads (w/o dressing)							
House	164	6	2	7	9	21	360
Caesar	103	3	1	5	8	13	23
Chicken Caesar	183	6	2	37	19	15	286
Chinese Chicken	421	13	3	35	24	56	472
BBQ Chicken	371	17	9	96	33	23	559
Sides (hot)							
Baked Yams	198	0	0	0	3	47	14
Black Beans	209	3	1	0	12	34	851
Butternut Squash	99	0	0	0	2	26	8
Creamed Spinach	99	6	2	7	4	10	567
Green Beans	58	3	2	6	2	8	129
Hand Mashed Potatoes	185	5	3	15	3	32	362
Homemade Stuffin	161	10	5	23	4	17	4307
Hot Potatoes	129	3	1	4	2	24	133
Kernel Corn	103	0	0	0	4	26	211
Macaroni & Cheese	312	11	6	25	15	25	813
Roasted Garlic Potatoes	145	3	1	4	3	28	204
Saffron Rice	159	3	1.5	6	3	30	295
Steamed Vegetables	35	0	0	0	2	7	28
Sides (cold)							
Cucumber Salad	30	0	0	0	1	7	109
Creamy Cole Slaw	237	20	4	28	1	14	637
Tangy Tomato Salad	46	3	0	0	1	6	348
Soups							
Ten Vegetable Soup	121	3	0	0	3	21	620
Turkey Dumpling Soup	166	4	1	54	19	14	890
Extras							
Balsamic Vinaigrette	60	4	1	54	19	14	890
BBQ Dressing	45	2	0.5	0	0	6	242
Caesar Dressing	170	19	3	15	0	1	180
Chinese Chicken Salad Dressing	100	8	1	0	0	8	105
Cranberry sauce	45	0	0	0	0	11	14
Gravy	94	9	3	9	0.3	3	240
Lavash (flatbread)	60	0	0	0	3	12	90
Roll, 1/2	150	1.5	0.3	0	6	29	310

Item	Calories	Fat (g)	Sat. fat (g)	Cholesterol (mg)	Protein (g)	Carbs (g)	Sodium (mg)
McDonald's							
Breakfast							
Egg McMuffin	300	12	4.5	235	18	29	830
Sausage McMuffin	370	23	8	45	14	28	790
Sausage McMuffin With Egg	450	28	10	255	20	29	930
English Muffin	150	2	0.5	0	5	27	260
Sausage Biscuit	410	28	8	35	10	30	930
Sausage Biscuit with Egg	490	33	10	245	16	31	1010
Bacon, Egg & Cheese Biscuit	480	31	10	250	20	31	1410
Biscuit	240	11	2.5	0	4	30	640
Ham and Egg Cheese Bagel	550	23	8	255	26	58	1490
Spanish Omelet Bagel	690	38	14	275	27	60	1570
Steak and Egg Cheese Bagel	700	35	13	290	38	57	1290
Sausage	170	16	5	35	6	0	290
Scrambled Eggs (2)	160	11	3.5	425	13	1	170
Hash Browns	130	8	1.5	0	1	14	330
Hotcakes (Plain)	340	8	1.5	20	9	58	630
Hotcakes (Margarine 2 pats & Syrup)	600	17	3	20	9	104	770
Breakfast Burrito	290	16	6	170	13	24	680
Sandwiches							
Hamburger	280	10	4	30	12	35	590
Cheeseburger	330	14	6	45	15	36	830
Quarter Pounder	430	21	8	70	23	37	840
Quarter Pounder with Cheese	530	30	13	95	28	38	1310
Big Mac	590	34	11	85	24	47	1090
Big N' Tasty	540	32	10	80	24	39	970
Big N' Tasty with Cheese	590	37	12	95	27	40	1210
Crispy Chicken	500	26	4.5	50	22	46	1100
Filet-O-Fish	470	26	5	50	15	45	890
Chicken McGrill	400	47	3	60	25	37	890
Chicken McGrill (plain w/o mayo)	300	6	1.5	50	24	37	800
French Fries							
Small	210	10	2.3	0	3	26	135
Medium	450	22	4	0	6	57	290
Large	540	26	4.5	0	8	68	350
Super Size	610	29	5	0	9	77	390

Item	Calories	Fat (g)	Sat. fat (g)	Cholesterol (mg)	Protein (g)	Carbs (g)	Sodium (mg)
Chicken McNuggets							
Chicken McNuggets (4p)	210	13	2.5	35	10	12	460
Chicken McNuggets (6p)	310	20	4	50	15	18	680
Chicken McNuggets (9p)	460	29	6	75	22	27	1020
Condiments							
Hot Mustard Sauce (1 pkg)	60	3.5	0	5	1	7	240
Barbeque Sauce (1 pkg)	45	0	0	0	0	10	250
Sweet 'N Sour Sauce (1 pkg)	50	0	0	0	0	11	140
Honey (1 pkg)	45	0	0	0	0	12	0
Honey Mustard (1 pkg)	50	4.5	0.5	10	0	3	85
Light Mayonnaise (1 pkg)	45	4.5	0.5	10	0	1	100
Salad							
Chef Salad	150	8	3.5	95	1	5	740
Garden Salad	100	6	3	75	7	4	120
Grilled Chicken Caesar Salad	100	2.5	1.5	40	17	3	240
Salad Dressings							
Caesar (1 pkg)	150	13	0	10	1	5	400
Fat Free Herb Vinaigrette (1 pkg)	35	0	1.5	0	0	8	260
Honey Mustard (1 pkg)	160	11	2.5	15	1	13	260
Ranch (1 pkg)	170	18	1	15	0	3	460
Red French Reduced Calorie (1 pkg)	130	6	1	0	0	18	360
1000 Island (1 pkg)	130	9	1.5	15	1	11	350
Muffins/ Danish							
Low fat Apple Bran Muffin	300	3	0.5	0	6	61	380
Apple Danish	340	15	3	20	5	47	340
Cheese Danish	400	21	5	40	7	45	400
Cinnamon Roll	390	18	5	65	6	50	310
Desserts							
Fruit 'n Yogurt Parfait	380	5	2	15	10	76	240
Fruit 'n Yogurt Parfait (w/o granola)	280	4	2	15	8	53	115
Vanilla Reduced Fat Ice Cream Cone	150	4.5	3	20	4	23	75
Strawberry Sundae	290	7	5	30	7	50	95
Hot Caramel Sundae	360	10	6	35	7	61	180
Hot Fudge Sundae	340	12	9	30	8	52	170

Item	Calories	Fat (g)	Sat. fat (g)	Cholesterol (mg)	Protein (g)	Carbs (g)	Sodium (mg)
Desserts							
Nuts (on sundaes)	40	3.5	0	0	2	2	55
Butterfinger McFlurry	620	22	14	70	16	90	260
M&M McFlurry	630	23	15	75	16	90	210
Nestle Crunch McFlurry	630	24	16	75	16	89	230
Oreo McFlurry	570	20	12	70	15	82	280
Baked Apple Pie	260	13	3.5	0	3	34	200
Chocolate Chip Cookie (1 pkg.)	280	14	8	40	3	37	170
McDonaldland Cookies (1 pkg.)	230	8	2	0	3	38	250
Triple Thick Shakes (16 fl. oz.)							
Vanilla	570	16	11	65	14	89	400
Chocolate	580	17	11	65	15	94	280
Strawberry	560	16	11	65	14	89	190
Kid's Treat Menu							
Danimal Drinkable Low-Fat Yogurt, Strawberry Explosion	90	1.5	1	5	4	16	55
Fruit Roll-Ups, Strawberry Sensation	50	1	0	0	0	12	55
Go-Gurt, Ronald's Strawberry Splash	70	2	1	5	2	11	40
Beverages							
1% Milk (8 fl. oz.)	100	2.5	1.5	10	8	13	115
Orange juice (16 fl. oz.)	180	0	0	0	3	42	5
Hi-C Orange Drink, small	160	0	0	0	0	44	30
Pizza Hut							
Medium Pizza, Hand-Tossed Crust (1 slice)							
Cheese	240	10	5	10	12	28	650
Pepperoni	280	13	6	20	13	28	790
Ham	250	10	5	20	14	28	800
Beef	330	17	8	25	16	29	880
Pork	320	16	7	25	16	29	920
Sausage	340	18	8	30	16	28	910
Supreme	270	12	5	20	13	29	730
Super Supreme	290	14	6	25	13	29	850
Meat Lover's	320	17	7	30	14	28	900
Veggie Lover's	220	8	3	5	9	29	580
Pepperoni Lover's	250	11	4.5	15	11	27	730
Chicken Supreme	230	7	3.5	15	13	29	650
Medium Pizza, Thin 'n Crispy Crust (1 slice)							
Cheese	200	9	5	10	10	22	590
Pepperoni	190	9	4	15	9	21	610

Item	Calories	Fat (g)	Sat. fat (g)	Cholesterol (mg)	Protein (g)	Carbs (g)	Sodium (mg)
Ham	170	7	3.5	15	9	21	610
Beef	270	15	7	25	13	22	750
Pork	270	14	6	25	13	22	820
Sausage	290	17	7	30	12	22	800
Supreme	250	13	6	20	12	23	710
Super Supreme	280	15	6	25	13	23	840
Meat Lover's	310	19	8	35	14	22	910
Veggie Lover's	190	7	3	5	8	24	520
Pepperoni Lover's	250	13	6	20	12	22	760
Chicken Supreme	200	7	3.5	20	12	23	620
Medium Pan Pizza (1 slice)							
Cheese	290	14	6	10	12	28	590
Pepperoni	280	14	5	15	11	28	610
Ham	260	12	4	15	11	28	610
Beef	330	18	7	20	14	29	690
Pork	320	17	6	20	13	29	730
Sausage	340	20	7	25	13	29	720
Supreme	320	17	6	20	13	29	670
Super Supreme	340	18	6	25	14	30	780
Meat Lover's	360	21	7	30	14	29	840
Veggie Lover's	270	12	4	5	10	30	510
Pepperoni Lover's	330	18	7	20	14	29	760
Chicken Supreme	270	12	4	15	13	29	580
Personal Pan Pizza (1 pizza)							
Cheese	630	28	12	25	28	71	1,370
Pepperoni	620	28	11	30	26	70	1,430
Ham	580	23	9	35	27	70	1,450
Beef	710	35	14	45	31	71	1,580
Pork	700	34	13	40	31	71	1,670
Sausage	740	39	14	55	31	71	1,640
Big New Yorker Pizza (1 slice)							
Cheese	410	18	9	20	20	46	1,210
Pepperoni	390	17	7	20	18	46	1,210
Ham	370	14	6	25	19	46	1,220
Beef	500	26	11	40	25	47	1,450
Pork	490	25	10	35	24	47	1,540
Sausage	530	29	12	50	24	47	1,510
Supreme	470	23	10	35	23	48	1,410
Veggie Lover's	480	22	6	10	19	57	1,410
Stuffed Crust Pizza (1 slice)							
Cheese	360	16	8	25	18	39	1,090
Pepperoni	360	16	7	30	17	39	1,120
Beef	390	18	8	30	19	40	1,150

Item	Calories	Fat (g)	Sat. fat (g)	Cholesterol (mg)	Protein (g)	Carbs (g)	Sodium (mg)
Stuffed Crust Pizza (1 slice) (continued)							
Pork	380	18	8	30	19	40	1,190
Sausage	400	20	8	35	19	40	1,180
Ham	330	13	6	30	18	39	1,130
Supreme	410	20	9	35	20	41	1,220
Super Supreme	340	18	6	20	13	32	780
Chicken Supreme	270	11	4	15	12	32	620
Veggie Lover's	270	11	4	5	9	33	550
Meat Lover's	350	19	7	25	14	31	830
Pepperoni Lover's	320	16	7	20	13	31	780
The Edge Pizza (1 slice)							
Veggie	70	3	1.5	< 5	4	9	180
Chicken Veggie	90	3.5	1.5	15	7	9	290
Meaty	160	11	4.5	20	7	8	440
Works	110	6	2.5	10	5	9	270
The Insider (1 slice)							
Cheese	370	16	8	30	17	41	890
Twisted Crust Pizza (1 slice)							
Cheese	450	16	8	15	20	58	1,210
Pepperoni	440	15	6	20	18	58	1,230
Supreme	470	18	8	25	20	59	1,280
1/2 P'zone (1 slice)							
P'zone Classic	200	34	60	7	15	25	42
P'zone Pepperoni	180	31	55	7	10	24	44
P'zone Meaty	270	48	75	13	15	24	57
Subway							
7 Under 6 low-fat 6" subs and delis							
Veggie Delite	200	2.5	0.5	0	7	37	500
Turkey Breast	254	3.5	1	20	16	39	1,000
Turkey Breast & Ham	267	4.5	1	26	18	40	1,210
Ham	261	4.5	1.5	25	17	39	1,260
Roast Beef	264	4.5	1	20	18	39	850
Subway Club	294	5	1.5	33	22	40	1,250
Roast Chicken Breast	311	6	1.5	48	25	40	880
Turkey Breast Deli	200	3.5	1	13	12	31	700
Ham Deli	194	3.5	1	12	10	30	750
Roast Beef Deli	206	4	1	13	12	31	600
Subway Classic 6" subs and delis							
Tuna with light mayo	419	21	5	42	18	39	1,180
Seafood & Crab with light mayo	378	16	4.5	24	14	46	1,270
Italian BMT	453	24	8	56	21	40	1,740
Cold Cut Trio	415	20	7	57	19	40	1,670

Item	Calories	Fat (g)	Sat. fat (g)	Cholesterol (mg)	Protein (g)	Carbs (g)	Sodium (mg)
Subway Melt	384	15	5	44	22	40	1,710
Steak & Cheese	362	13	4.5	37	23	41	1,190
Meatball	501	25	10	56	23	46	1,350
Tuna Deli	309	15	4	26	12	31	810
6" Subway Select Subs							
Honey Mustard Turkey with Cucumbers	275	3.5	1	20	16	45	990
Caesar Italian BMT	531	32	10	66	22	41	1,840
Horseradish Steak & Cheese	468	22	6	44	23	43	1,110
Southwest Chicken	362	13	2.5	44	21	40	960
Honey Mustard Melt	376	11	5	44	22	47	1,590
Asiago Caesar Chicken	391	15	3	47	22	41	1,000
Southwest Steak & Cheese	412	18	6	44	23	42	1,120
Wraps							
Asiago Caesar Chicken	413	15	3	47	22	47	1,320
Steak & Cheese	353	9	4	37	22	46	1,400
Turkey Breast & Bacon	321	7	2.5	28	18	45	1,510
Cookies							
Chocolate Chip	209	10	3.5	12	3	29	135
Oatmeal Raisin	197	8	2	14	3	29	175
Peanut Butter	220	12	3	0	3	26	200
M&M	210	10	3	13	2	29	135
White Chocolate Macadamia Nut	221	12	3	13	2	27	140
Sugar	222	12	3	18	2	28	170
Chocolate Chunk	210	10	3	12	2	30	150
7 Under 6 Low-Fat Salads							
Veggie Delite	50	1	0	0	2	9	310
Turkey Breast	105	2	0.5	20	11	11	820
Turkey Breast & Ham	117	3	0.5	26	13	11	1,030
Ham	112	3	1	25	11	11	1,070
Roast Beef	114	3	0.5	20	12	11	660
Subway Club	145	3.5	1	30	17	12	1,080
Roast Chicken Breast	137	3	0.5	36	16	12	730
Subway Classic Salads							
Tuna with light mayo	238	16	4	42	13	11	880
Seafood & Crab with light mayo	198	11	3.5	24	9	17	970
Italian BMT	273	19	7	56	16	11	1,440
Cold Cut Trio	234	15	6	57	14	11	1,370
Subway Melt	203	10	4.5	41	17	12	1,410
Steak & Cheese	182	8	3.5	37	17	12	890
Meatball	320	20	9	56	18	18	1,050

Item	Calories	Fat (g)	Sat. fat (g)	Cholesterol (mg)	Protein (g)	Carbs (g)	Sodium (mg)
Bread							
6" Italian	178	2	0.5	0	7	33	350
6" Wheat	186	1.5	0.5	0	7	36	360
6" Parmesan Oregano	195	3	1	4	8	34	400
6" Country Wheat	206	2.5	0.5	0	8	39	360
6" Hearty Italian	191	2	0.5	0	7	36	350
6" Asiago Cheese	220	5	3	8	9	34	460
6" Sourdough	265	3	1.5	0	10	49	460
Deli Style Roll	150	2.5	0.5	0	5	27	260
Wrap	200	2	0.5	0	0	45	720
Condiments							
Vinegar (1 tsp.)	1	0	0	0	0	0	0
Mustard (2 tsp.)	8	0	0	0	0	0	115
Light mayonnaise (1 tbsp.)	46	5	1	7	0	1	100
Mayonnaise (1 tbsp.)	111	12	3	9	0	0	80
Olive oil blend (1 tsp.)	45	5	1	0	0	0	0
Bacon (2 strips)	45	4	1.5	8	2	0	180
Fat-free dressings							
Italian	50	0	0	0	0	4	610
Ranch	60	0	0	0	1	14	530
French	70	0	0	0	0	17	390
Sauces							
Honey Mustard	28	0	0	0	0	7	140
Southwest	86	9	1.5	7	0	2	190
Horseradish	142	13	2	7	0	3	180
Asiago Caesar	110	11	2	10	1	2	230
Cheese (2 slices)							
Processed American cheese	41	3.5	2	10	2	0	200
Provolone cheese	51	4	2	11	4	0	125
Swiss cheese	53	4	2.5	13	4	0	30
Processed pepper jack cheese	40	3.5	2	11	2	0	210
Cheddar cheese	60	5	3	15	4	0	95
Taco Bell							
Tacos							
Taco	170	10	4	30	9	12	330
Taco Supreme	210	14	6	40	9	14	350
Soft Taco, Beef	210	10	4	30	11	20	570
Soft Taco, Chicken	190	7	2.5	35	13	19	480
Tacos							
Soft Taco, Steak	190	7	3	25	14	18	490
Soft Taco Supreme, Beef	260	13	6	40	11	22	590

Item	Calories	Fat (g)	Sat. fat (g)	Cholesterol (mg)	Protein (g)	Carbs (g)	Sodium (mg)
Soft Taco Supreme, Chicken	240	11	5	45	14	21	490
Soft Taco Supreme, Steak	240	11	5	35	15	20	510
Double Decker Taco	330	15	5	30	14	37	740
Double Decker Taco Supreme	380	18	7	40	15	39	760
Gorditas							
Gorditas Supreme, Beef	300	14	5	35	17	27	550
Gorditas Supreme, Chicken	300	13	5	45	16	28	530
Gorditas Supreme, Steak	300	14	5	35	17	27	550
Gorditas Baja, Beef	360	21	5	35	13	29	810
Gorditas Baja, Chicken	340	18	4	40	16	28	710
Gorditas Baja, Steak	340	18	4	30	17	27	730
Gorditas Nacho Cheese, Beef	310	15	4	25	13	30	780
Gorditas Nacho Cheese, Chicken	290	13	2.5	25	15	29	690
Gorditas Nacho Cheese, Steak	290	13	3	20	16	28	700
Gorditas Santa Fe, Beef	380	23	5	35	14	31	700
Gorditas Santa Fe, Chicken	370	20	4	40	17	30	610
Gorditas Santa Fe, Steak	370	20	4.5	35	17	29	620
Chalupas							
Chalupas Supreme, Beef	380	23	8	40	14	29	580
Chalupas Supreme, Chicken	360	20	7	45	17	28	490
Chalupas Supreme, Steak	360	20	7	35	17	27	500
Chalupas Baja, Beef	420	27	7	35	14	30	760
Chalupas Baja, Chicken	400	24	5	40	17	28	660
Chalupas Baja, Steak	400	24	6	30	17	27	680
Chalupas Nacho Cheese, Beef	370	22	6	25	13	30	740
Chalupas Nacho Cheese, Chicken	350	19	4.5	25	16	29	640
Chalupas Nacho Cheese, Steak	350	19	4.5	20	16	28	660
Chalupas Santa Fe, Beef	440	29	7	35	14	31	660
Chalupas Santa Fe, Chicken	420	26	6	40	17	30	560
Chalupas Santa Fe, Steak	430	27	6	35	18	29	580
Burritos							
Bean Burrito	370	12	3.5	10	13	54	1,080
7-Layer Burrito	520	22	7	25	16	65	1,270

Item	Calories	Fat (g)	Sat. fat (g)	Cholesterol (mg)	Protein (g)	Carbs (g)	Sodium (mg)
Burritos (continued)							
Chili Cheese Burrito	330	13	5	25	13	40	900
Burrito Supreme, Beef	430	18	7	40	17	50	1,210
Burrito Supreme, Chicken	410	16	6	45	20	49	1,120
Burrito Supreme, Steak	420	16	6	35	21	48	1,140
Double Burrito Supreme, Beef	510	23	9	60	23	52	1,500
Double Burrito Supreme, Chicken	460	17	6	70	27	50	1,200
Double Burrito Supreme, Steak	470	18	7	55	28	48	1,230
Fiesta Burritos, Beef	380	15	5	30	14	49	1,100
Fiesta Burritos, Chicken	370	12	3.5	35	17	48	1,000
Fiesta Burritos, Steak	370	12	4	25	18	47	1,020
Specialties							
Tostada	250	12	4.5	15	10	27	640
Mexican Pizza	390	25	8	45	18	28	930
Enchirito, Beef	370	19	9	50	18	33	1,300
Enchirito, Chicken	350	16	8	55	21	32	1,210
Enchirito, Steak	350	16	8	45	22	31	1,220
MexiMelt	290	15	7	45	15	22	830
Taco Salad With Salsa	850	52	14	70	30	69	2,250
Taco Salad With Salsa, no shell	400	22	10	70	24	31	1,510
Cheese Quesadilla	350	18	9	50	16	31	860
Chicken Quesadilla	400	19	9	75	25	33	1,050
Nachos and sides							
Nachos	320	18	4	< 5	5	34	560
Nachos Supreme	440	24	7	35	14	44	800
Nachos Bell Grande	760	39	11	35	20	33	1,300
Mucho Grande Nachos	1,320	82	25	75	31	116	2,670
Pintos 'n Cheese	180	8	4	15	9	18	640
Mexican Rice	190	9	3.5	15	5	23	750
Cinnamon Twists	150	4.5	1	0	1	27	190
Condiments							
Border Sauce, Mild	0	0	0	0	0	0	60
Border Sauce, Hot	0	0	0	0	0	0	80
Border Sauce, Fire	0	0	2.5	0	0	0	100
Picante Sauce	0	0	0	0	0	1	110
Red Sauce	10	0	0	0	0	2	220
Condiments							
Green Sauce	5	0	0	0	0	1	150
Nacho Cheese Sauce	120	10	2.5	5	2	5	470

Item	Calories	Fat (g)	Sat. fat (g)	Cholesterol (mg)	Protein (g)	Carbs (g)	Sodium (mg)
Pepper Jack Cheese Sauce	70	7	1	5	0	1	120
Santa Fe Sauce	100	10	1.5	10	0	1	75
Fiesta Sauce	5	0	0	0	0	1	55
Southwest Sauce	20	0	0	0	< 1	3	15
Sour Cream	40	4	2.5	10	1	1	10
Guacamole	35	3	0	0	0	1	80
Cheddar Cheese	30	2	1.5	5	2	0	45
Three Cheese Blend	25	2	1	5	2	0	60
Togo's							
Sandwiches							
California Roasted Chicken Sandwich	510	15	N/A	65	36	73.2	1,768
Ham & Cheese Sandwich	660.8	26	N/A	68	33.3	76	2,900
Turkey and Cheese Sandwich	638	22.5	N/A	71	34	75	2,277
Turkey and Cranberry Sandwich	623	13.5	N/A	49	30	96	1,904
Meatball with Pizza Sauce, Produce, & Parmesan Sandwich	707	28	N/A	97	36	78.2	1,602
Hot or Cold Roast Beef Sandwich	552	11.3	N/A	84.3	42.4	72.6	1,536
Hot Pastrami	705	26.5	N/A	72	33.6	85	2,260
Pastrami Reuben Sandwich	875	44.5	N/A	111	43.6	85	2,460
Hummus Sandwich	668	21	N/A	9	19.5	102	1,510
Italian Dry, Salami, Capicolla, Mortadella, Cotto & Provolone Sandwich	736	32	N/A	85	31	74	2,191
Egg Salad with Cheese Sandwich	728	35	N/A	456	29	76	1,765
Albacore Tuna Sandwich	701	29.5	N/A	67	32	78	1,653
Swiss, American, Provolone Cheese Sandwich	859	45.5	N/A	107	42	77	2,196
Italian Dry Salami & Cheese Sandwich	770	33	N/A	118	42	78	3,288
Avocado & Turkey Sandwich	675	28	N/A	35	27	80	1,606
Bar-B-Q Beef	724	21.5	N/A	88	39	94	2,120
Turkey & Ham with Cheese Sandwich	670	25	N/A	760	37	76	2,772
Avocado, Cucumber, & Alfalfa Sprouts Sandwich	637	28	N/A	6	16	85	1,150

Item	Calories	Fat (g)	Sat. fat (g)	Cholesterol (mg)	Protein (g)	Carbs (g)	Sodium (mg)
Sandwiches (continued)							
Chunky Chicken Salad Sandwich	636	26	N/A	42	40	72	1,562
Turkey & Bacon Club Sandwich	667	26	N/A	813	37	73	21,082
Salads							
Taco Salad	943	59	N/A	71	29	76	1,623
Garden Salad	226	10	N/A	216	12	31	579
Chef Salad	387	19.5	N/A	655	265	26	15,866
Oriental Salad	499	21	N/A	41	25	49	1,062
Caesar Salad	471	30	N/A	72	30	23	1,189
Potato Salad	215	13	N/A	11	2	25	435
Condiments							
Blue Cheese Dressing	291	30.2	N/A	20.1	2	3	662.8
Thousand Island	231	222	N/A	30	1	9	532
Ranch	321	33	N/A	15	2	5	64
Reduced-Calorie Italian	60	4.5	N/A	0	0	4	693
Oriental	221	14	N/A	5	0	24	512
Caesar	241	23	N/A	20	2	8	633
Sweet & Spicy	70	0	N/A	0	0	19	703
Reduced-Calorie Ranch	1,901	16	N/A	25	1	10	603
Wendy's							
Sandwiches							
Classic Single with everything	410	19	7	70	24	37	890
Big Bacon Classic	570	29	12	100	34	46	1,460
Jr. Hamburger	270	9	3	30	14	34	600
Jr. Cheeseburger	310	12	5	45	17	34	820
Jr. Bacon Cheeseburger	380	18	7	55	20	34	890
Jr. Cheeseburger Deluxe	350	16	6	45	17	37	890
Hamburger, Kid's Meal	270	9	3	30	14	33	600
Cheeseburger, Kid's Meal	310	12	5	45	17	34	820
Grilled Chicken Sandwich	300	7	1.5	55	24	36	740
Chicken Breast Fillet Sandwich	430	16	3	55	27	46	750
Chicken Club Sandwich	470	19	4	65	30	47	920
Spicy Chicken Sandwich	430	15	3	60	27	47	1,240
Garden Sensation Salads							
Caesar Side Salad	70	4	2	15	7	2	250
Side Salad	35	0	0	0	2	7	20
Chicken BLT Salad	310	16	8	60	33	10	1,100
Mandarin Chicken	150	1.5	0	10	20	17	650
Spring Mix Salad	180	11	6	30	11	12	230
Taco Supremo Salad	360	17	9	65	27	29	1,090

Item	Calories	Fat (g)	Sat. fat (g)	Cholesterol (mg)	Protein (g)	Carbs (g)	Sodium (mg)
Condiments							
Homestyle Garlic Croutons	70	2.5	0	0	1	9	120
Caesar Dressing	150	16	2.5	20	1	1	240
Honey Mustard Dressing	310	29	4.5	25	1	12	410
Roasted Almonds	130	12	1	0	4	4	70
Crispy Rice Noodles	60	2	0.5	0	1	10	180
Oriental Sesame Dressing	280	21	3	0	2	21	620
Honey Roasted Pecans	130	13	1	0	2	5	65
House Vinaigrette Dressing	220	20	3	0	0	9	830
Taco Chips	220	11	2	0	3	25	150
Sour Cream	60	6	3.5	15	1	1	15
Salsa	30	0	0	0	1	6	440
Blue Cheese Dressing	290	30	6	45	2	3	870
Creamy Ranch	250	25	4	15	1	5	640
Fat-Free French Style	90	0	0	0	0	21	240
Low-Fat Honey Mustard	120	3.5	0	0	0	23	370
Reduced-Fat Creamy Ranch	110	9	1.5	15	1	7	610
French fries							
Kid's Meal	250	11	2	0	3	36	220
Medium	390	17	3	0	4	56	340
Biggie	440	19	3.5	0	5	63	380
Great Biggie	530	23	4.5	0	6	75	450
Hot Stuffed Baked Potatoes							
Plain	310	0	0	0	7	72	25
Bacon & Cheese	580	22	6	40	18	79	950
Broccoli & Cheese	480	14	3	5	9	81	510
Sour Cream & Chives	370	6	4	15	7	73	40
Country Crock Spread	60	7	1.5	0	0	0	115
Chili							
Small	200	6	2.5	35	17	21	870
Large	300	9	3.5	50	25	31	1,310
Cheddar cheese, shredded	70	6	3.5	15	4	1	110
Saltine Crackers	25	0.5	0	0	1	4	80
Hot Chili Seasoning	5	0	0	0	0	2	280
Crispy Chicken Nuggets							
5 pieces	220	14	3	35	11	13	480
4 pieces (Kid's Meal)	180	11	2.5	25	9	10	380
Barbecue Sauce	40	0	0	0	1	10	160
Honey Mustard Sauce	130	12	2	10	0	6	210
Sweet & Sour Sauce	45	0	0	0	0	12	115

Item	Calories	Fat (g)	Sat. fat (g)	Cholesterol (mg)	Protein (g)	Carbs (g)	Sodium (mg)
Frosty							
Junior, 6 oz.	170	4	2.5	20	4	28	100
Small, 12 oz.	330	8	5	35	8	56	200
Medium, 16 oz.	440	11	7	50	11	73	260

APPENDIX B:
Useful Nutrition Resources

Airlines

Alaska Airlines	www.alaskaair.com
America West Airlines	www.americawest.com
American Airlines	www.aa.com
Continental Airlines	www.continental.com
Delta Air Lines	www.delta.com
JetBlue	www.jetblue.com
Northwest Airlines	www.nwa.com
Southwest Airlines	www.southwest.com
United Airlines	www.united.com
US Airways	www.usairways.com

Fast Food Companies

Arby's	www.arby.com
Baja Fresh	www.bajafresh.com
Blimpie	www.blimpie.com
Boston Market	www.bostonmarket.com
Burger King	www.burgerking.com
Carl's Jr	www.burgers.com
Chick-Fil-A	www.chickfila.com
Del Taco	www.deltaco.com
Domino's	www.dominos.com
El Pollo Loco	www.elpolloloco.com
Hardee's	www.hardees.com
In-N-Out	www.in-n-out.com
Jack in the Box	www.jackinthebox.com
Jamba Juice	www.jambajuice.com
Kentucky Fried Chicken	www.kfc.com
Koo Koo Roo	www.kookooroo.com
McDonald's	www.mcdonalds.com
Noah's Bagels	www.noahs.com

Pizza Hut	www.pizzahut.com
Quizno's Subs	www.quiznos.com
Subway	www.subway.com
Taco Bell	www.tacobell.com
Togo's	www.togos.com
Wendy's	www.wendys.com

Hotel Chains

Doubletree	www.doubletree.com
Embassy Suites	www.embassysuites.com
Four Seasons	www.fourseasons.com
Hilton	www.hilton.com
Holiday Inn	www.holiday-inn.com
Hyatt	www.hyatt.com
Marriott	www.marriott.com
Radisson	www.radisson.com
Ritz Carlton	www.ritzcarlton.com
Sheraton	www.sheraton.com

Additional Resources

National Restaurant Association
www.restaurant.org

National Institutes of Health
Office of Dietary Supplements
www.ods.od.nih.gov/index.aspx

BIBLIOGRAPHY

Introduction

Weinstein, E. Help I'm Drowning in E-Mail. *The Wall Street Journal*. January 10, 2002.

Chapter 1

Mayes, Frances. 1997. Under the Tuscan Sun. New York: Broadway Books.

Chapter 2

Arnold, L.M., et al. Effect of isoenergetic intake of three or nine meals on plasma lipoproteins and glucose metabolism. *American Journal of Clinical Nutrition*, 1993; 57(3):446-451.

Benton, D., et al. The influence of breakfast and a snack on psychological functioning. *Physiology and Behavior*, 2001; 74(4-5):559-571.

Connor, W.E., and Bendich, A. (eds.). Highly unsaturated fatty acids in nutrition and disease prevention. *American Journal of Clinical Nutrition*, 2000; 71(Suppl.):169s-398s.

Drummond, S., et al. A critique of the effects of snacking on body weight status. *European Journal of Clinical Nutrition*, 1996; 50(12):779-783.

Edelstein, S., et al. Increased meal frequency associated with decreased cholesterol concentrations: Rancho Bernardo, CA, 1984-1987. *American Journal of Clinical Nutrition*, 1993; 55(3):664-669.

Gatenby, S. Eating frequency: Methodological and dietary aspects. *British Journal of Nutrition*, 1997; 77(Suppl. 1):S7-S20.

Hanks, W.A., et al. An examination of coping strategies used to combat driver fatigue. *Journal of American College of Health*, 1999; 48(3):135-137.

Jenkins, D.J., et al. Nibbling versus gorging: Metabolic advantages of increased meal frequency. *New England Journal of Medicine*, 1989; 321(14):929-934.

Jenkins, D.J., et al. Metabolic advantages of spreading the nutrient load: Effects of increased meal frequency in non-insulin-dependent diabetes. *American Journal of Clinical Nutrition*, 1992; 55(2):461-467.

Jenkins, D.J., et al. Implications of altering the rate of carbohydrate absorption from the gastrointestinal tract. *Clinical and Investigative Medicine*, 1995; 18(4):296-302.

Jenkins, D.J.A., et al. Effect of nibbling versus gorging on cardiovascular risk factors: Serum uric acid and blood lipids. *Metabolism*, 1995; 44(4):549-555.

Jones, P.J.H., et al. Meal-frequency effects on plasma hormone concentrations and cholesterol synthesis in humans. *American Journal of Clinical Nutrition*, 1993; 57(6):868-874.

Kanarek, R.B., and Swinney, D. Effects of food snacks on cognitive performance in male college students. *Appetite*, 1990; 14(1):15-27.

Kirk, T.R. Role of dietary carbohydrate and frequent eating in body-weight control. *Proceedings of the Nutrition Society*, 2000; 59(3):349-358.

McGrath, S.A., and Gibney, M.J. The effects of altered frequency of eating on plasma lipids in free-living healthy males on normal self-selected diets. *European Journal of Clinical Nutrition*, 1994; 48:402-407.

Oliver, G., and Wardle, J. Perceived effects of stress on food choice. *Physiology and Behavior,* 1999; 66(3):511-515.

Powell, J.T., et al. Does nibbling or grazing protect the peripheral arteries from atherosclerosis? *Journal of Cardiovascular Risk,* 1999; 6(1):19-22.

Westerterp-Plantegna, M.S., et al. Food intake in the daily environment after energy-reduced lunch, related to habitual meal frequency. *Appetite,* 1994; 22:173-182.

Wyatt, H.R., et al. Long-term weight loss and breakfast in subjects in the National Weight Control Registry. *Obesity Research,* 2002; 10(2):78-82.

Chapter 3

Food Marketing Institute (FMI's) trends in the United States—Consumer attitudes and the super-market. 2000. FMI:Washington, DC

U.S. Food and Drug Administration. *The new food label.* HFI-40. Rockville, MD: U.S. Food and Drug Administration, 1994.

Chapter 4

Biing-Hwan, L., and Frazao, E. *Away-from-home foods increasingly important to quality of American diet.* Agriculture Information Bulletin No. 749. Washington, DC: Economic Research Service, USDA, January 1999.

Borrud, L.G. Eating out in America: Impact on food choices and nutrient profiles. Available at www.barc.usda.gov/bhnrc/foodsurvey/Eatout95.html. Accessed February 15, 2003.

Clemens, L.H.E., et al. The effect of eating out on quality of diet in premenopausal women. *Journal of the American Dietetic Association,* 1999; 99:442-444.

Frazao, E. (ed.). *America's eating habits: Changes and consequences.* Agriculture Information Bulletin No. 750. Washington, DC: Economic Research Service, USDA, 1999.

Jacobson, M.F., and Hurley, J. *Restaurant confidential.* New York: Workman, 2002.

Jones-Mueller, A., et al. *Healthy dining in Los Angeles restaurant nutrition guide,* 4th ed. San Diego, CA: Healthy Dining Publications, 2002. Available at www.healthy-dining.com. Accessed February 15, 2003.

Lichten, J.V. *Dining lean.* Houston: Nutrifit, 2000.

Natow, A.B., and Heslin, J. *Eating out food counter.* New York: Pocket Books, 1998.

Warshaw, H. *The restaurant companion.* Chicago: Surrey Books, 2nd ed. 1995.

Webb, D. *International cuisines calorie counter.* New York: M. Evans, 1990.

Chapter 6

Physicians Committee for Responsible Medicine. Airport food ratings 2002. Available at www.pcrm.org/news/health021113report.html. Accessed July 21, 2003.

Chapter 7

Associated Press (London). Dieting said to impair memory. October 13, 1995.

Cowen, P.J., et al. Why is dieting so difficult? *Nature,* 1995; 376:557.

Cowen, P.J., et al. Moderate dieting causes a 5-HT2c receptor supersensitivity. *Psychological Medicine*, 1996; 26:1155-1159.

Daee, A. Psychologic and physiologic effects of dieting in adolescents. *Southern Medical Journal*, 2002; 95(9):1032-1041.

Editorial staff. Obesity: The numbers. *Nutrition Today*, 2002; 37(6):224.

Field, A.E., and Colditz, G.A. Frequent dieting and the development of obesity among children and adolescents. *Nutrition*, 2001; 17(4):355-356.

Food and Nutrition Board, Institute of Medicine. *Dietary reference intakes for energy, carbohydrates, fiber, fat, fatty acids, cholesterol, protein and amino acids.* Washington, DC: National Academy Press, 2002.

Kassirer, J.P., and Angell, M. Losing weight, an ill-fated New Year's resolution. *New England Journal of Medicine*, 1998; 338(1):52-54.

Medscape Wire. Unrealistic weight loss goals result in feelings of failure. November 13, 2000. www.medscape.com/viewarticle/412245

National Eating Disorders Association. www.nationaleatingdisorders.org.

Oliver, G., and Wardle, J. Perceived effects of stress on food choice. *Physiology and Behavior*, 1999; 66(3):511-515.

Reidel, W.J., et al. Tryptophan, mood, and cognitive function. *Brain, Behavior, and Immunity*, 2002; 16:581-589.

Roth, G. *Breaking free from compulsive eating.* 1984 (p.37). Bobbs-Merrill: New York.

St. Jeor, S.T., et al. Dietary protein and weight reduction. A statement for healthcare professionals from the Nutrition Committee of the Council on Nutrition, Physical Activity and Metabolism of the American Heart Association. *Circulation*, 2001; 104:1869-1874.

Teixeira, P.J., et al. Weight loss readiness in middle-aged women: Psychosocial predictors of success for behavioral weight reduction. *Journal of Behavioral Medicine*, 2002; 25(6): 499-523.

Tribole, E., and Resch, E. *Intuitive eating*, 2nd ed. New York: St. Martin's Press, 2003.

U.S. Department of Agriculture. Dieting can slow reaction time. *Food and Nutrition Research Briefs*, 1997; April:1.

Chapter 8

American Cancer Society. The complete guide—Nutrition and physical activity. Available at www.cancer.org/docroot/PED/content/PED_3_2X_Diet_and_Activity_Factors_That_ Affect_Risks.asp?sitearea=COM. Accessed October 13, 2002.

Anderson, J.W. *Plant fiber in foods*, 2nd ed. Lexington, KY: HCF Nutrition Research Foundation, 1990.

Appel, L.J., et al. A clinical trial of the effects of dietary patterns on blood pressure. *New England Journal of Medicine*, 1997; 336(16):1117-1124.

Expert Panel on Detection, Evaluation, and Treatment of High Blood Cholesterol in Adults. Executive summary of the third report of the National Cholesterol Education Program (NCEP) Expert Panel on Detection, Evaluation, and Treatment of High Blood Cholesterol in Adults (Adult Treatment Panel III). *Journal of the American Medical Association*, 2001; 285:2486-2497.

Food and Nutrition Board, Institute of Medicine. *Dietary reference intakes for energy, carbohydrates, fiber, fat, fatty acids, cholesterol, protein and amino acids.* Washington, DC: National Academy Press, 2002.

Frazao, E., ed. The high costs of poor eating patterns in the United States. *America's eating habits: Changes and consequences.* Agriculture Information Bulletin, No. 750. Washington, DC: Economic Research Service, USDA, 1999.

Howard, B.V., and Wylie-Rosett, J. AHA scientific statement: Sugar and cardiovascular disease—A statement for healthcare professionals from the Committee on Nutrition of the Council on Nutrition, Physical Activity, and Metabolism of the American Heart Association. *Circulation*, 2002; 106:523-527.

Krause, R.M., et al. AHA scientific statement: AHA dietary guidelines revision 2000: A statement for healthcare professionals from the Nutrition Committee of the American Heart Association. *Circulation*, 2000; 102:2296-2311.

National Institutes of Health (NIH). *NIH consensus statement: Optimal calcium intake.* 12(4), 1994. http://consensus.nih.gov/cons/097/097_intro.htm

National Institutes of Health (NIH). The Dash Diet. NIH publication no. 98-4082. Washington, DC: May 2001.

The Surgeon General's report on nutrition and health. DHHS (PHS) publication no. 88-50210. Washington, DC: U.S. Department of Health and Human Services, 1988.

U.S. Departments of Agriculture and Health and Human Services. *The food guide pyramid.* USDA Home and Garden Bulletin No. 249. Washington, DC: U.S. Departments of Agriculture and Health and Human Services, 1992.

U.S. Departments of Agriculture and Health and Human Services. *Dietary guidelines for Americans,* 5th ed. USDA Home and Garden Bulletin No. 232. Washington, DC: USDA, 2000.

U.S. Department of Health and Human Services. *Healthy people 2010,* 2nd ed. 2 vols. Washington, DC: U.S. Government Printing Office, November 2000. Available at www.health.gov/healthypeople. Accessed October 15, 2002.

Vollmer, W.M., et al. Effects of diet and sodium intake on blood pressure: Subgroup analysis of the DASH-Sodium Trial. *Annals of Internal Medicine,* 2001; 135:1019-1028.

Whelton, P.K., et al. Primary prevention of hypertension: Clinical and public health advisory from the National High Blood Pressure Education Program. *Journal of the American Medical Association,* 2002; 288(15):1882-1888.

Wilson, P.W., et al. Prediction of coronary heart disease using risk factor categories. *Circulation,* 1998; 97:1837-1847.

World Cancer Research Fund, American Institute for Cancer Research. *Food, nutrition and the prevention of cancer: A global perspective.* Washington, DC: World Cancer Research Fund, 1997.

Chapter 9

Brown, B.G., et al. Simvastatin and niacin, antioxidant vitamins, or the combination for the prevention of coronary disease. *New England Journal of Medicine,* 2001; 345:1583-1592.

Devaney, B., and Barr, S. DRI, EAR, RDA, AI, UL—Making sense of this alphabet soup. *Nutrition Today,* 2002; 37(6):226-232.

Fairfield, K.M., and Fletcher, R.H. Vitamins for chronic disease prevention in adults: Scientific review. *Journal of the American Medical Association,* 2002; 287(23):3116-3126.

Fletcher, R.H., and Fairfield, K.M. Vitamins for chronic disease prevention in adults: Clinical applications. *Journal of the American Medical Association,* 2002; 287(23):3127-3129.

Food and Nutrition Board, Institute of Medicine. *Dietary reference intakes for vitamin A, vitamin K, arsenic, boron, chromium, copper, iodine, iron, manganese, molybdenum, nickel, silicon, vanadium, and zinc.* Washington, DC: National Academy Press, 2001.

Hunt, J. Commentary: Tailoring advice on dietary supplements: An opportunity for dietetic professionals. *Journal of the American Dietetic Association*, 2002; 102(12):1754-1755.

Liebman, B. Antioxidants no magic bullet. *Nutrition Action Health Letter*, 2002; 29(2):1-8.

Omenn, G.S., et al. Effects of a combination of beta carotene and vitamin A on lung cancer and cardiovascular disease. *New England Journal of Medicine*, 1996; 334:1150-1155.

Position of the American Dietetic Association: Food fortification and dietary supplements. *Journal of the American Dietetic Association*, 2001; 101(1):115-125.

Sarubin, A. *The health professional's guide to popular dietary supplements*. Chicago: American Dietetic Association, 2000.

Trumbo, P., et al. Commentary: Dietary reference intakes: Dietary reference intakes for vitamin A, vitamin K, arsenic, boron, chromium, copper, iodine, iron, manganese, molybdenum, nickel, silicon, vanadium, and zinc. *Journal of the American Dietetic Association*, 2001;101(3) 294-301.

Tufts University. From our research labs: You can't always take it in pill form. *Health and Nutrition Letter*, 2002; 20(10):3.

U.S. Food and Drug Administration. Tips for the savvy supplement user: Making informed decisions and evaluating information. Available at www.cfsan.fda.gov/~dms/ds-savvy.html. Accessed January 2002.

Chapter 10

Birch, L.L. Children's food acceptance patterns. *Nutrition Today*, 1996; 31(6):234-240.

Daee, A. Psychologic and physiologic effects of dieting in adolescents. *Southern Medical Journal*, 2002; 95(9):1032-1041.

Fisher, J.O., and Birch, L.L. Restricting access to palatable foods affects children's behavioral response, food selection, and intake. *American Journal of Clinical Nutrition*, 1999; 69:1264-1272.

Fisher, J.O., and Birch, L.L. Parent's restrictive feeding practices are associated with young girls' negative self-evaluation of eating. *Journal of the American Dietetic Association*, 2000; 100:1341-1346.

Fisher, J.O., and Birch, L.L. Eating in the absence of hunger and overweight in girls from 5 to 7 y of age. *American Journal of Clinical Nutrition*, 2002; 76:226-231.

Gillman, M.W., et al. Family dinner and diet quality among older children and adolescents. *Archives of Family Medicine*, 2000; 9:235-240.

Leung, S., and Vranica, S. Happy Meals are no longer bringing in smiles at McDonald's. *Wall Street Journal*, January 31, 2003, p. B1.

Rampersaud, G.C., et al. National survey beverage consumption data for children and adolescents indicate the need to encourage a shift toward more nutritive beverages. *Journal of the American Dietetic Association*, 2003; 103:97-100.

Rolls, B.J., et al. Serving portion size influences 5-year-old but not 3-year-old children's food intakes. *Journal of the American Dietetic Association*, 2000; 100:232-234.

Siega-Riz, A.N., et al. Trends in breakfast consumption for children in the United States from 1965 to 1991. *American Journal of Clinical Nutrition*, 1998; 67(Suppl.):748s-756s.

Society for Nutrition Education. Guidelines for childhood obesity prevention programs: Promoting healthy weight in children. October 2002. Available at www.sne.org. Accessed December 2002.

Chapter 11

American College of Sports Medicine, American Dietetic Association, and Dietitians of Canada. Joint position statement: Nutrition and athletic performance. *Medicine and Science in Sports and Exercise,* 2000; 32(12):2130-2145.

Bennardot, D. *Nutrition for serious athletes.* Champaign, IL: Human Kinetics, 2000.

Clark, N. *Nancy Clark's sports nutrition guidebook,* 2nd ed. Champaign, IL: Human Kinetics, 1997.

Costill, D.L. Carbohydrates for exercise: Dietary demands for optimal performance. *International Journal of Sports Medicine,* 1988; 9:5.

Food and Nutrition Board, Institute of Medicine. *Dietary reference intakes for energy, carbohydrates, fiber, fat, fatty acids, cholesterol, protein and amino acids.* Washington, DC: National Academy Press, 2002.

Foster-Powell, K., et al. International table of glycemic index and glycemic load values. *American Journal of Clinical Nutrition,* 2002; 76:5-56.

Jenkins, D.J.A., et al. Glycemic index: Overview of implications in health and disease. *American Journal of Clinical Nutrition,* 2002; 76:266s-273s.

Ludwig, D.S., and Eckel R.H. The glycemic index at 20 y. *American Journal of Clinical Nutrition,* 2002; 76:264s-265s.

Martin, W.R., and Fuller, R.E. Suspected chromium picolinate–induced rhabdomyolysis. *Pharmacotherapy,* 1998; 18(4):860-862.

Jellin, J.M., Gregory P.J., Batz F., Hitchens K., et al. *Pharmacist's Letter-Prescriber's Letter Natural Medicine Comprehensive Database,* 4th ed. Stockton, CA: Therapeutic Research Faculty, 2002

Sherman, W. Carbohydrates, muscle glycogen, and muscle glycogen supercompensation. In: Williams, M.H., ed. *Ergogenic aids in sport,* p. 13. Champaign, IL: Human Kinetics, 1983.

Skinner, R., et al. Ergogenic aids. In: Rosenbloom, C.A., ed. *Sports nutrition: A guide for the professional working with active people,* pp. 107-146. Chicago: American Dietetic Association, 2000.

Chapter 14

Yanovski, J.A., et al. A prospective study of holiday weight gain. *New England Journal of Medicine,* 2000; 342:861-867.

INDEX

ABOUT THE AUTHOR

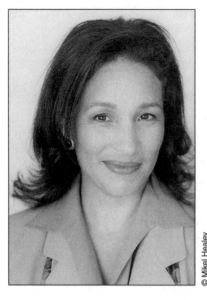

© Mikel Healey

Evelyn Tribole is a registered dietitian who operates a private practice counseling athletes, executives, families, and other groups on the art of eating healthy in spite of a hectic lifestyle. An expert whom millions have turned to, Tribole was the nutritionist for "Good Morning America" and has appeared frequently in the national media. Currently she is the nutritionist for Lifetimetv.com.

Tribole conducts nutrition workshops nationwide for both national and local groups and has written many books including the first two editions of *Eating on the Run*, *Healthy Homestyle Cooking* (over 900,000 copies in print), and *Healthy Homestyle Desserts*.

Tribole earned a master's degree in nutrition science from California State University at Long Beach. She has received the Excellence in Private Practice award from the American Dietetic Association and is also an accomplished runner who qualified for the Olympic marathon trials in 1984.

Tribole lives in Irvine, California.